T0178796

PRAISE FOR *100 ESSENTIAL ANSWERS TO YOUR ORTHODONTIC QUESTIONS*

"Dr. Chung provides great insight into the orthodontic specialty, a real behind-the-scenes look. I would highly recommend this book to both dental professionals and patients alike. A must read for anyone interested in orthodontic treatment."

—Dr. Leonid Epshteyn, Nanuet, New York

"A complete guide you must read before getting braces. Dr. Chung explains the orthodontic treatment as if he is explaining it to his family and friends. Very easy to follow and will answer all of your questions. Highly recommended."

—Dr. Sung H. Lee, Edgewater, New Jersey

"Do you really want the truth about orthodontics? Then rush to read Dr. Christopher H. Chung's new book. Written in a breezy, conversational style and well organized in a question-and-answer format, this book will equip you to make the decision to undergo orthodontic treatment for you or your children. Dr. Chung himself is a superb, thoughtful, and skilled practitioner."

—Dr. Michael G. Steinberg, Short Hills, New Jersey

"This is a must-read book for those who are thinking about getting braces. The information contained in the book is invaluable, and you won't find it elsewhere. If nothing else, read the section about fees—it is eye opening. Highly recommended."

—Dr. Richard H. Shin, Oradell, New Jersey

100 ESSENTIAL ANSWERS TO YOUR ORTHODONTIC QUESTIONS

100
ESSENTIAL
ANSWERS

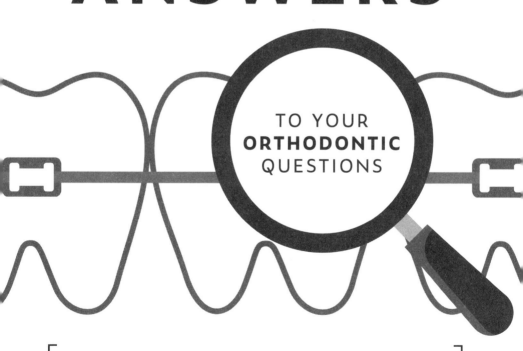

TO YOUR
ORTHODONTIC
QUESTIONS

[DR. CHRISTOPHER H. CHUNG]

Advantage.

Published by Advantage, Charleston, South Carolina.
Member of Advantage Media Group.

ADVANTAGE is a registered trademark, and the Advantage colophon is a trademark of Advantage Media Group, Inc.

Printed in the United States of America.

10 9 8 7 6 5 4 3 2 1

ISBN: 978-1-64225-118-0
LCCN: 2020911604

Cover design by Mary Hamilton.
Layout design by Megan Elger.

This publication is designed to provide accurate and authoritative information in regard to the subject matter covered. It is sold with the understanding that the publisher is not engaged in rendering legal, accounting, or other professional services. If legal advice or other expert assistance is required, the services of a competent professional person should be sought.

Advantage Media Group is proud to be a part of the Tree Neutral® program. Tree Neutral offsets the number of trees consumed in the production and printing of this book by taking proactive steps such as planting trees in direct proportion to the number of trees used to print books. To learn more about Tree Neutral, please visit www.treeneutral.com.

Advantage Media Group is a publisher of business, self-improvement, and professional development books and online learning. We help entrepreneurs, business leaders, and professionals share their Stories, Passion, and Knowledge to help others Learn & Grow. Do you have a manuscript or book idea that you would like us to consider for publishing? Please visit advantagefamily.com or call 1.866.775.1696.

To my loving wife, Laura,
and my two beautiful daughters, Katie and Lauren.

ACKNOWLEDGMENTS

I want to thank Katie, my daughter, for taking time out of her busy schedule to draw the illustrations.

CONTENTS

Common Questions

1. How is an orthodontist different from a regular dentist? Aren't they pretty much the same? I've heard dentists do braces too, so why wouldn't I just get the dentist I already see to fix my teeth?

2. Now that I'm ready to get braces, how can I find an orthodontist I can really trust? Since there are so many of them, how would I know I've chosen the right one?

3. I've never understood how braces work, and I'm curious about it since I'd like to get my teeth fixed soon. How is it possible to move my teeth without breaking them? Aren't they attached to solid bone?

4. My teeth aren't that crooked, so I was surprised when I went to see an orthodontist and found out that fixing them would take a lot longer than I expected. Why would straightening a few teeth take so long?

5. I just want my teeth to look straight, but my orthodontist says my bite needs to be corrected too. I don't care about my bite. So why should I bother getting it fixed? Can't I just ask him to fix my teeth?

6. Isn't there some way to speed up treatment time for my kids? If not, how long does it usually take to have teenagers' teeth straightened?

7. Can you explain in detail how braces are put on teeth? I just want to know what to expect. Is it done during a single appointment, or does it take several? Is it a painful process?

8. How long do I have to wait to eat after getting braces? Will it hurt when I chew, and do I

have to avoid certain foods at first?

9. What should I do if I need to get braces but I don't have a regular dentist? Don't I need a referral from a dentist to see an orthodontist?

10. After seeing three orthodontists for a free consultation, each prescribed a different treatment approach to straighten my teeth. How do I know which practitioner or recommendation is best?

11. It's embarrassing to ask, but I want to know if it's safe to kiss my girlfriend who has braces too. Can't my own braces get stuck to her braces and wires if I kiss her?

12. When I need to fly, I'm afraid my new braces will set off the metal detectors as I go through security at the airport. Has that actually happened to anyone?

13. Seeing how the orthodontist was able to change my teeth and give me a different smile was really interesting. Even though I'm only seventeen, I'm now seriously considering becoming an orthodontist in the future. What would I need to do?

Preteen Phase-One Early Treatment

14. Our orthodontist says my nine-year-old daughter needs to be older before she gets braces, but most of her friends already have theirs. Why do some children get braces earlier? She's complaining about having to wait, and we're wondering why we can't get her braces now. Do we really have to postpone treatment?

15. When is the best time to get my son braces? Should I wait to see an orthodontist until he's lost all of his baby teeth and his permanent teeth have already come in?

16. I have a ten-year-old daughter who recently went to see an orthodontist for an exam and x-ray. The orthodontist advised us to have a few of her baby teeth removed. Since baby teeth will naturally fall out, why do these need to be taken out at all? Wouldn't her baby teeth naturally fall out on their own?

17. What should I do when my son is still sucking his thumb as an eight-year-old? We've tried everything to break the habit, but nothing seems to work. Can you suggest something to help him stop? I'm worried it will make his teeth crooked. Is that true?

18. Some of my child's eight-year-old friends already have expanders, but I have no idea how they work. What are they, and why are they needed? Will getting or wearing an expander hurt?

19. A dentist just told me my seven-year-old son's upper front teeth are sticking out

because his lower jaw is positioned too far back, and he'll eventually need jaw surgery to fix it. Is there anything else we can do?

20. Are underbites genetic? Is there anything I can do to keep one from getting worse? My seven-year-old daughter seems to have an underbite like me, and I'm worried she's going to have a jutting chin that sticks out and jaw pain like I do. Will braces help, or will she need jaw surgery to fix this?

21. Can I stay with my daughter during her orthodontic visits, since I already do that when she goes to the dentist? Do you ever need to use antianxiety medication when you treat kids the way some dentists do for dental procedures?

22. Since my child's teeth aren't crooked, why would she need braces? Aren't braces just for people who want straight teeth?

23. I've made an appointment for my kids to see an orthodontist, but he wants to have x-rays taken as part of their exam. I'm concerned about exposing my children to radiation, so I'd like to skip the x-rays. Is this kind of imaging really necessary?

24. My eight-year-old daughter needs a space maintainer, and I was told an impression mold of her teeth has to be made. But she has a strong gag reflex. She's worried she may throw up when the molding material is in her mouth. She's scared and doesn't want to go to her appointment. What can I do?

CHAPTER 3 . . . . **41**

Teen Treatment

25. Our dentist says my twelve-year-old daughter is ready for braces, and she's scheduled her for a consultation with an orthodontist. I'm just curious about what will happen during that consultation, and if she's ready, will my daughter get braces the same day? How long will it take to put her braces on? Doesn't it usually take a few hours?

26. After taking my teenage daughter to an orthodontist for an examination and x-rays, he told me one of her canine teeth is stuck high on her upper jaw. I'm upset because he says she needs to see an oral surgeon to try to save the tooth, but she might need an implant if he can't. What do you think I should do?

27. I'm the parent of a thirteen-year-old who will be needing braces soon. But I hated my braces as a kid, and I don't want my son to go through what I did. Are they as miserable as I remember?

28. Although my fourteen-year-old son had his braces removed six months ago, his teeth

have become crooked again. When we went back to see the orthodontist, he told us we'd need to start over with braces. Do you think we made a mistake and got our son's braces put on too early when he was twelve? Should we have waited until he was fourteen or fifteen before starting orthodontic treatment?

29. Do your teen patients ever talk about being made fun of? I'm worried my daughter is going to get bullied for her braces. I know kids get ridiculed for wearing glasses, so won't that happen to kids wearing braces too?

30. As a parent, I want all the information I can get about how braces could affect my teen's health. Are there any risk factors to wearing braces? What are the pros and cons? Do the benefits outweigh any potential risks?

31. I know a lot has changed since I had braces as a child, and I'd like to have my daughter benefit from the newest orthodontic treatment available for kids. Which is the one you recommend most highly, and why do you think it's the best?

32. I'm worried about my son getting cavities and stains while wearing braces. Are there special mouth rinses and other products my son can use to keep his braces clean and strengthen his enamel? Which ones do you recommend? Would he be expected to brush his teeth at school?

33. Now that my son has braces, we keep having to go back to his orthodontist because they keep coming loose. Is this normal?

34. My teen daughter swallowed one of her brackets today. She's not really concerned and doesn't have any symptoms. What should I do?

35. Even though my teenage son is the right age to get braces, he absolutely refuses to get them. He wants Invisalign because it doesn't show. Is Invisalign a good option for kids? Does it work as well as braces?

36. Since my son's teeth are very crowded and crooked, there doesn't seem to be enough room in his mouth for all of them. I'm afraid some of his permanent teeth will have to be removed. Is there any way to avoid that?

37. Will getting braces hurt my daughter's ability to play her flute? Can she still play a wind instrument while she's wearing braces?

38. We have an appointment with an orthodontist to get braces for our son, who is active in sports. Will he be able to continue playing football and basketball with braces on? Could this make him more prone to getting injuries?

39. Can getting braces negatively affect my fifteen-year-old in any way? Will it keep her from completing schoolwork or cause her to miss school? Since my daughter is an honor

student, I'm worried getting braces will hurt her grades. And what about meals and snacks? Can she still eat candy and drink juice?

Adult Treatment

40. Many years ago, my dentist told me I needed braces for my bite issues. I never got treatment back then, but I think I'm finally ready to start braces even though I'm fifty-eight. Am I too old to get them? Is there anything I need to do first?

41. Is it okay for me to get braces if I'm pregnant? I still want to get my teeth fixed, but would you advise I wait or go ahead with it?

42. Someone just told me I can get my teeth fixed right away with instant orthodontics and veneers without having to wait a year for results like I would with regular braces. Since I have a gap and need to get my teeth straightened, are these good options for me?

43. What are lingual braces? I've heard they're impossible to see when someone has them. If that's the case, why wouldn't everyone get them? Are they a good option instead of metal braces? Am I a candidate?

44. I'm trying to decide whether to get Invisalign or braces. I don't really prefer either one. What are the pros and cons?

45. When I got Invisalign, the orthodontist put a lot of little bumps on my teeth, and I don't like them. I thought Invisalign was supposed to be totally invisible. Why do I need to have these little nodules stuck to my teeth?

46. I really don't want to get braces, period! I don't even want to have clear braces, but I've heard good things about Invisalign. How would it work if I opted to try it to straighten my teeth?

47. As a twenty-eight-year-old guy, I'm embarrassed to admit dental procedures make me nervous, but I really need to get my teeth fixed. My wife makes fun of me because I'm afraid to get braces if it means I'll have to deal with needles and shots as part of the treatment. Are there any braces I could get that don't cause any sort of pain?

48. After a consultation with one orthodontist, I was told my case is too complex and that he wouldn't feel comfortable treating me with Invisalign. I went for a second opinion and was told that I'm definitely a candidate for Invisalign. What gives? How do I know which of them is right?

49. My job requires me to talk constantly. Will it be harder to speak clearly once I have

braces on? Will my speech be affected in any way?

50. Since I'm a professional singer, I'm worried about braces ruining my career. Will braces affect my singing?

51. Because I have a dental phobia, I'm scared of needles. Will you be using needles if I come in to get braces? And do you need to take impressions of my teeth? I once threw up in the middle of that process, and I gag when I have to bite into dental film. Can I avoid any of this?

52. Even though I had braces when I was young, I can see my lower teeth shifting and getting crooked again. My upper teeth are still pretty straight. So can I just get braces for the bottom ones?

53. Would it be okay to have my family dentist fit me with braces, since he says he can do it? Can I get the same result if he does my orthodontic work, or do I need to see an orthodontist? What's the difference between a dentist and an orthodontist anyway?

54. Can I still get braces even though I have some crowns, root canals, and fillings? I also have some missing teeth. But I've always wanted to get my teeth straightened. Can you still do it?

Fees and Insurance

55. How much will treatment cost? I'd like to get braces, but I'm wondering if I can actually afford them. Can you give me some idea of what people usually pay?

56. What does an orthodontist's fee typically cover? I went in for a free consultation and got an estimate for the cost of my braces treatment. But will the fee I was quoted cover everything from beginning to end?

57. I have three children who need braces, and I want them for myself too. But I'm not sure if I can afford it. Will my dental insurance cover the cost of orthodontic treatment, or should I try to sign up for an additional insurance policy to cover it?

58. Since I never had braces as a kid, my teeth are gradually getting worse. I'm finally ready to get treatment for myself, but I'm not sure if I can afford it. Can I pay for my braces with a payment plan, or do I need to pay everything in full?

59. Without calling a lot of orthodontists, how do I know I'm not being overcharged to get my teeth fixed?

60. After I went to see an orthodontist and got a quote for fixing my teeth, I found a second

doctor who gave me a much lower quote. Why would there be such a big difference? And why pay more if I can get my teeth straightened more affordably by an orthodontist who will do the work for less?

61. I'm thinking about getting Invisalign because I don't want to wear braces that show. Is Invisalign a lot more expensive than braces?

62. What happens if I move in the middle of my child's orthodontic treatments? I want to start their braces soon, since it's about the right time. But we may be moving to another state in about eight months. Would I get a refund for the fees I've already paid?

63. My son started Invisalign treatment about four months ago, but his treatment isn't going well because he's not wearing the trays like he's supposed to. I'm thinking we will have to switch over to braces. I'm scared of having to start all over again. What do you think I should do?

64. Unfortunately, I lost my retainer at college and stopped wearing it for a few months. I haven't had a chance to go back to my orthodontist yet, and now I'm worried because I've noticed my teeth have shifted. Will I need to get braces all over again?

65. Is it okay to try to negotiate a reduction in the cost of my orthodontic treatment? How can I qualify to get the maximum discount? Is there a time or season I should start treatment to get the best deal?

Technology

66. Are today's braces better than the ones people had twenty years ago? If so, how will my sixth-grade son with an overbite benefit from advances in braces technology?

67. As a young career woman in my twenties, I don't want braces. What other new orthodontic technologies are available to me if I decide to get my teeth fixed?

68. My college friends keep talking about how happy they are wearing Invisalign instead of braces, and I'm thinking about getting my teeth fixed too. Can you explain how Invisalign works? And what would I have to do to start using it?

69. I'm a mom of three kids who need braces, but they want Invisalign instead because that's what their friends have. Does Invisalign treatment take longer than traditional braces? Is it okay for all ages?

70. When I go online, I keep seeing offers for mail-order aligner treatment. Is this an option that's as safe and effective as getting Invisalign through an orthodontist?

71. Since I'm getting married in eight months, I want to start and finish my braces within that time period. Is there a way to accelerate my treatment? If so, are there any risks to doing it faster?

72. Can accelerated orthodontic treatment harm my children's teeth in any way? Won't moving teeth too fast cause serious problems?

73. My coworker told me about SureSmile technology, but she didn't tell me what it is or how it works. Can you explain how this technology is different from normal braces and how it can benefit me when I get braces?

74. Although I understand how SureSmile works, I don't want to pay more for my daughter's braces. Why should I pay extra when regular braces will give her the same results?

75. Is it worth it to try to find an orthodontist who is using the new 3D x-ray machines? Can 3D imaging really help my family's orthodontic treatments have a better outcome than 2D imaging?

76. Radiation exposure from 3D x-rays is a big concern for me, so I don't want to have a CT taken for braces treatment. Is my concern justified or not?

77. I don't like having molding material in my mouth because it makes me gag, so I'm relieved to hear some orthodontists are using a new kind of impressionless scanning. Does this kind of scanner emit radiation?

Nontraditional Treatment

78. Will orthodontic treatment help with mouth breathing? I've noticed my child has a hard time breathing through his nose, and he's constantly walking around with his mouth open. Won't that predispose him to having more cavities since it dries out his mouth?

79. Can orthodontic treatment help my sleep apnea get better or go away completely? My doctor referred me to an orthodontist after telling me I have the condition, but how is sleep apnea related to my teeth?

80. Since my daughter snores, I'm worried that's a sign she may have an airway obstruction. Can braces help with this?

81. I was told that sleep apneas can sometimes lead to symptoms of ADHD in children. I've also heard that orthodontic treatment can help improve ADHD behaviors. Is this true?

82. My orthodontist said I need jaw surgery. But when I went for a second opinion, I was told that I can be treated with miniscrews instead of surgery. What is miniscrew treatment,

and how does it work?

83. Do you think my severe headaches could be linked to my bad bite? I've tried everything, but nothing seems to be working, and sometimes I can barely stand the pain at my job. Could orthodontic treatment help?

84. My daughter's jaws make a popping sound when she opens her mouth, and she says there's a place just below her ear that's started hurting. Could this be a problem orthodontics could relieve, and if not, is it likely to get worse as she gets older?

85. Our thirteen-year-old son has been grinding his teeth in his sleep since childhood, and we'd like to know if braces can fix the problem, since we know it can damage his teeth long term. If not, do you recommend we have a custom night guard made for him, or can he use an over-the-counter night guard?

86. After a little more than two years in braces, I just got my braces off. I'm excited to be finished, and my teeth are straight, but I'm not completely happy about how I look. I think my gums have changed and are covering too much of my teeth, and I'd like to have that fixed. Is there any way to do that?

87. Now that my braces are off, I was advised to have my wisdom teeth taken out, even though they're healthy, so my teeth will stay straight. I don't even know which teeth they are, and if they're not decayed, why would they have to be extracted?

88. When my orthodontist prescribed Invisalign therapy, he advised I use remote Dental Monitoring because I'm a nurse who has little time off. Can you explain how remote monitoring works and how it will help me while I'm getting my teeth fixed with Invisalign?

Post-braces: What to Expect

89. What exactly is a retainer, and why will I have to wear one? I'm a high school senior who's just graduated and had my braces taken off. I wanted to be finished with wearing braces before I start college next fall, but now I've been told I'll have to wear a retainer. Are there different types of retainers with different benefits? Which one is best?

90. As a busy working mom, I don't have time to research the pros and cons of which retainer is best for my teen who is about to get her braces off. Since there are different types of retainers, which one should I get for my daughter and why?

91. Working as a computer programmer, I have a lot of deadlines, and I forgot to wear my retainer for two weeks while I was finishing a software project. Now I'm worried because I

can see that my teeth have shifted, and my retainer is hard to get on and doesn't seem to fit like it used to. What should I do?

92. My teenage son just got his braces off, but he seems confused about how to take care of his retainer. As a single dad, I don't want to have to micromanage this task, so I'd like to know what you consider the most important best-use retainer guidelines my son will need to follow when using his retainer at home and school. Are there precautions he will need to take that he should know about?

93. Now that I've had my clear retainers for about a year, I just noticed my retainer is cracking, especially in the back. Since it's hard to take time off from my job to see my orthodontist, I'd like to know if this is normal. Is it okay to keep using it? Or should I call my orthodontist and order a replacement retainer?

94. How long will my retainers last? Since I live in a rural area an hour's drive from my orthodontist, I was wondering if I'll have to replace them anytime soon. Will I have to get new ones in the future, or can I keep using the ones I was just given when my braces were taken off?

95. I'm about to get married, and I was excited to have my braces taken off before the ceremony. But now I see white spots on my teeth, and I'm concerned since they weren't there before I got braces. What are these discolorations, and why do I have them? Is there some way to make them go away quickly?

96. Should I have my wisdom teeth removed? I had braces a few years ago, but now I think my lower front teeth are shifting forward. Could my wisdom teeth be the cause?

97. After I got married, I found out my husband didn't like me wearing my retainers at night. I can wear them when he's not around, but I'd prefer not to have to wear them at all. When can I stop wearing retainers?

98. Does everyone need to wear retainers after they get their braces off, or am I a special case for some reason? My coworkers say my teeth look great, now that my teeth are fixed. But my orthodontist says I'll still need to wear a retainer. Is this really necessary, and if so, how long will I have to use it?

99. I understand why I have to wear a retainer, but the one I was given has metal bands and large, pink plastic sections. My friends wear smaller retainers that look like clear trays, so why did I get different ones? I've also heard about permanent retainers. What are they, and would they work better for me for some reason?

100. With myself and two kids in braces, I'm concerned about the cost of replacing our retainers once our treatments are done. How long are retainers supposed to last? I know

we'll have to wear them long term, so can you tell me how to help my kids and me take care of them, so I don't have to replace them too frequently?

INTRODUCTION

H ello! I'm Dr. Christopher H. Chung, and if you're reading this book, I know you're someone who already has braces or is thinking about getting them for yourself or your children. I also know you must have a lot of questions about braces and how they might change your daily life. That's why I've written this book. It provides the essential knowledge keys you'll need to make the very best choices about orthodontic treatment for yourself and your children. Whatever your unique circumstances, you can find the vital, need-based information you're seeking in an easy-to-access question-and-answer format you can put to use right away. This format enables you to personalize your information search quickly and easily, so you won't have to wade through pages of information that aren't applicable to your individual situation.

The book's question-and-answer format was intentionally chosen to grant you easy access to the expert information I share with my patients in my own orthodontic practice every day. Based on more than twenty years of experience in orthodontics, my answers provide the essential information you need to make the right decisions along your treatment path. When it comes to getting braces, knowledge is power, just as it is in every other venture. And I'm delighted to give you the vital knowledge you need to make the most well-informed decisions about your orthodontic treatment. While doing so, I also explain what orthodontics is and why it's so important to your overall physical and emotional health.

As a specialist in orthodontics, I've spent the last two decades giving patients of all ages new *healthy* smiles. I don't simply straighten teeth so they look good cosmetically. I'm also trained to detect and correct any underlying bite problems that might negatively affect my patients' teeth and jaw functions. This is especially important for children, because early detection and treatment of their bite issues at a young age is critical to preventing the need for corrective jaw surgery later in their lives. So even though I know creating a beautiful smile is important, fixing a bad bite is vital too. Doing so can prevent the development of lifelong chronic pain and jaw malfunction that may negatively affect a person's ability to eat or talk normally. And because I've stayed on the cutting edge of the most recent orthodontic innovations, I'm able to fix my patients' bites and align their teeth more quickly and comfortably than ever before. In fact, for the last ten years, I've been one of the few elite providers offering patients the SureSmile robotic customized technique and "hidden" braces they can wear behind their teeth if they're seeking an alternative to either braces or Invisalign. Yet these are just two of the many different advances now available to adults and children needing straighter teeth and a better bite.

Orthodontists like me are seeing a steady transition away from traditional braces as more and more patients are choosing new treatments that can align their teeth faster and better than ever before. These effective nontraditional methods include self-litigating braces, lingual braces, and removable aligners like Invisalign. And their success has been fueled by the fact that these innovative braces and aligners not only look better cosmetically but provide faster results too. One of the reasons they actually work so well is because recent technological advances have created better diagnostic techniques and better control of the "anchors" I attach to teeth to move them. Another impetus to the rising popularity of these treatments is the growing number of men and women who are no longer embarrassed to seek orthodontic treatment as adults—thanks to the better aesthetic of hidden braces and Invisalign. In place of the braces, wires, and elastic bands of traditional braces, Invisalign straightens teeth via the use of clear, removable plastic tooth aligners. Many adults who were embarrassed to use metal braces to fix their teeth are suddenly eager to resolve orthodontic problems they'd resigned themselves to living with for the rest of their lives. And they no longer have to, now that better-looking options are available and affordable. Children, too, are finding the idea of invisible aligner trays to be far less frightening than a mouthful of metal braces. In other words, nontraditional approaches are proving invaluable to kids and grownups alike—whether they're sixteen or sixty.

I have so much more I'd like to tell you about the latest orthodontic technologies and techniques I use, and I'm sure you have a lot of questions you'd like to ask *me*. With all these new choices, you'll need to find out which technology will actually deliver the results you're striving for and which I recommend most highly to my own patients. You might want to know when you should start specific treatments for yourself or your child, how long each treatment will take, and what to expect from the treatment process itself. And if you are like most people, you're also probably wondering how much adjusting a person's teeth and bite is likely to cost and what financing options are available to pay for such treatment.

I can answer these questions, and many more besides, because I've been practicing orthodontics for so many years, and I've heard the same questions over and over again from my patients. Of course, I'm happy to answer my patients' questions about how to best fix their teeth and jaws during their visits, but I know there are thousands of others asking those same questions whom I may never meet personally. So I realized an "orthodontic answer book" was needed, one filled with my expert answers to questions you might typically ask before, during, and after treatment to straighten your teeth or align your jaw. But here's the problem: the average person *won't know what they don't know* about orthodontic treatment, and what they don't know can definitely hurt them. Waiting too long to bring in a child whose lower teeth have worn down because of a bad bite, for example, may mean it's too late to fix them. Similarly, my individual patients often neglect to ask me questions they never thought, or knew, to inquire about in the first place.

In other words, there's a lot of essential orthodontic information a nonspecialist simply won't have the knowledge base to reference. This book can help with that too. The following pages are filled with my expert recommendations as I answer the many multifaceted questions about braces and other treatments I've been sharing one on one with my patients as a practicing orthodontist for two decades. Although I've heard a lot of the same treatment-related questions over the years, every one of my patients is an individual with unique characteristics and concerns—just like you. And the answers I provide in this book reflect how my orthodontic knowledge has been applied to the various issues and circumstances you are likely to encounter in your own specific treatment-related scenarios.

Can you trust my expert advice? The accounts and success stories of real patients I share in the last chapter of this book will verify that you can, and my credentials speak for themselves. After graduating with a Doctor of Dental Surgery from the University of California, Los Angeles, I completed a three-year specialty program in orthodontics and obtained a Master of Science in oral biology from the University of Medicine and Dentistry of New Jersey (now Rutgers University). I also graduated from the Roth/Williams Center for Functional Occlusion, and my orthodontic practice reflects that institution's commitment to provide health-based treatment prioritizing a well-functioning bite that also looks good cosmetically. After all, you need your newly straightened teeth for both eating *and* smiling!

So whether you're an adult considering orthodontic treatment for the first time or a parent looking for expert guidance about how to best correct your child's bite and teeth, this book can help. I'll answer your questions about available treatment options, choosing a provider, pain concerns, cost worries, and more. Whatever questions you have about braces, or about orthodontics in general, you'll find the answers here—plus, you'll acquire a wealth of useful new knowledge you can apply right away. What's more, you don't need to read this book from front to back, starting with the very first page. Instead, you can use its nine sections as a topical guide to locate the specific questions and answers that uniquely pertain to you or your kids during each stage of braces treatment. But the book is so easy to pick up and read, you'll find many helpful answers to important questions you simply never thought to ask!

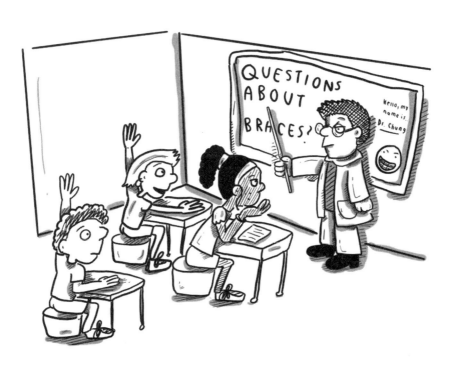

CHAPTER 1

COMMON QUESTIONS

T he following questions and answers reflect the topics my first-time patients ask me about most frequently when they're considering getting braces or other kinds of orthodontic treatment for themselves or their children. I've found that providing accurate answers to these common questions is the best way to resolve their concerns about what it's like for a person to have their teeth or jaws "fixed" and how it may affect their life. I want to do the same for you. In this chapter, I'll help inform your treatment decisions by explaining the difference between dentists and orthodontists and advise you about how to find an orthodontist you can really trust with reshaping your smile and correcting your bite. In addition, I'll describe how braces move teeth, what it's like to have braces put on, and how long this and other treatments may take. I'll also offer valuable insights about why it's so important to fix a bad bite, plus dispel a few common myths before explaining how a person becomes an orthodontist in the first place.

1. How is an orthodontist different from a regular dentist? Aren't they pretty much the same? I've heard dentists do braces too, so why wouldn't I just get the dentist I already see to fix my teeth?

Orthodontists acquire three years of additional training after graduating from dental school to specialize in straightening teeth and correcting bad bites. Thanks to all that extra training, orthodontists are specialists who typically limit their practice to providing treatments that align teeth and fix misaligned jaws. So they won't offer other regular dental services like filling cavities and cleaning teeth. If you hear of a general dentist who *does* provide orthodontic services, you can be certain that person isn't actually an orthodontist. And although these dentists may offer to do braces themselves, they won't have the extensive, specific knowledge and training needed to properly correct a person's jaw or align a person's teeth for life. Just like any other area of the medical field, dentistry has many specialties, and orthodontics is the one that focuses on fixing your bite and straightening your teeth with braces, Invisalign, and other treatment tools.

2. Now that I'm ready to get braces, how can I find an orthodontist I can really trust? Since there are so many of them, how would I know I've chosen the right one?

I'm glad you asked those crucial questions, since changing your orthodontist once you get braces can slow your progress or alter the results of your treatment. Here's a checklist to guide your search for a competent orthodontist you can trust for yourself or your child throughout the entire treatment process from start to finish:

- When looking for an orthodontist, it's wise to verify that any practitioner you're considering is actually an orthodontist as opposed to a general dentist. A family dentist simply won't have the specialized training in braces treatment, bite correction, and early intervention you're going to need.

> When looking for an orthodontist, it's wise to verify that any practitioner you're considering is actually an orthodontist as opposed to a general dentist.

- Another important factor to consider is an orthodontist's experience level, so you'll want to find out how many years they've been in practice. It's also important to ask how many cases like yours a practitioner has treated and request to see before and after photos of those types of patients.

- Of course, word-of-mouth recommendations for orthodontists are valuable too, especially if you know someone who's happy with their braces treatment and results. Likewise, it's a good idea to ask your general dentist to help you find an orthodontist, since dentists see the results of orthodontic treatment in so many of their own dental patients.

- And because you probably already use Google reviews or social media to assess other products and services, conducting an online search for information and patient feedback about different orthodontists makes a lot of sense too.

- If I were a patient, I would look for an established practice that's actually owned by an orthodontist and use that specialist (if everything else I've discussed checks out) instead of choosing an orthodontist who's just an employee at a practice. Why? Well, it's more likely a hired orthodontist will leave any given practice, and you may end up being treated by several different orthodontists over the course of your treatment. This isn't an ideal situation; it has downsides similar to building a house or completing a renovation project with several different contractors—you may not end up with the results you wanted or expected. You really should start and finish your braces treatment with the same orthodontist.

- I would also look for a practitioner who is not too young or too old. This is just my personal opinion, but I have good reasons to think this way. Someone who is too young probably just graduated and may not have the experience to treat complex cases. Believe me, I thought I knew everything when I first graduated as an orthodontist twenty years ago, but over time, and after treating thousands of cases, I've become a better orthodontist than I was when I started out. Having said that, I wouldn't choose an old orthodontist who's close to retiring either. Although it's not always the case, more senior orthodontists may not stay up to date with the newest orthodontic innovations and techniques, or their skills could have deteriorated over time due to age. So I advise finding someone with a few years of experience who still has many years of work ahead of them to ensure they're knowledgeable of and proficient in the latest orthodontic technologies.

- Lastly, you might assume orthodontists are all pretty much the same, but they're not. Just like any other doctor, some have better skills than others, and those varying skill levels may produce different results. I wouldn't choose an orthodontist based on price alone, just as I wouldn't buy the cheapest car I could find before going on a road trip. I think you'll agree this might not be the best approach.

---

3. I've never understood how braces work, and I'm curious about it since I'd like to get my teeth fixed soon. How is it possible to move my teeth without breaking them? Aren't they attached to solid bone?

The whole process of moving teeth *is* pretty amazing! Rather than applying a strong force to reposition your teeth, an orthodontist moves individual teeth by using a constant light pressure instead. The application of gentle constant force on a tooth is key to enabling that tooth to shift without being damaged. Orthodontists are trained to use a variety of different tools designed to exert the exact right amount of force needed to reposition your teeth most efficiently—without causing any harm to the tooth or the bone surrounding it.

This approach works well because your teeth aren't directly attached to the bone of your upper and lower jaws but to a soft layer of ligaments lying between your teeth and the underlying jawbone itself. When the gentle force of braces or Invisalign is applied, cells called *osteoclasts* remove bone, while cells called *osteoblasts* add bone. During this continuous dynamic process, the bone surrounding particular teeth is remodeled and reshaped as the force being applied slowly shifts teeth into their new positions. What this means is that an orthodontist is essentially moving and restructuring the bone in your jaws as they straighten your teeth. How cool is that?

4. My teeth aren't that crooked, so I was surprised when I went to see an orthodontist and found out that fixing them would take a lot longer than I expected. Why would straightening a few teeth take so long?

When you think of your teeth being straight or crooked, it's likely you're paying attention only to your front teeth. If those look pretty straight, you may assume you don't need much in the way of treatment. Most of my patients think that way when they first come in to see me. Like you, they're usually most concerned about the way their teeth *look* instead of how they physically *function* in their jaw. They don't realize they may have significant bite issues that need to be fixed to preserve their teeth and even their health. And despite what you might expect, it's usually more challenging to treat a patient with mostly straight teeth than it is to treat a patient with obviously crooked teeth. That's because better-looking teeth may mask a patient's bad bite, something that takes more time to fix than the crooked teeth of a patient with a proper bite.

Even though correcting a person's bite is more difficult and takes more time than just straightening teeth, it's more essential, because it has to do with function rather than aesthetics. Although aesthetics is certainly important, bite function is more crucial because it affects the overall *health* of your teeth and the jaw joint itself. Symptoms of bite problems are often so subtle and hard to detect they aren't easily noticed by anyone but a trained orthodontist. So don't be surprised if your orthodontist determines your case is more complex than you thought it would be. I would, however, advise you to get a second (or third) orthodontist's opinion to verify your original evaluation. If their opinions all concur or are pretty similar, you can be confident the treatment offered is correct.

5. I just want my teeth to look straight, but my orthodontist says my bite needs to be corrected too. I don't care about my bite. So why should I bother getting it fixed? Can't I just ask him to fix my teeth?

Having a good bite is important because a bad bite can lead to many health issues, including temporomandibular joint (TMJ) dysfunction or other jaw problems. Since your upper and lower teeth are meant to fit together properly when you chew, the TMJ is subjected to abnormal pressure when they don't. The resulting wear and tear of the joint's discs can lead to pain when the TMJ is opening and closing and even trigger locking of the jaw itself. Since a web of muscles wraps around the jaws and the TMJ, a bad bite may ultimately lead to persistent jaw pain and cause chronic headaches.

I've seen a lot of patients who lived with those dysfunctions for so long, they thought their symptoms were simply a normal part of life. Once their bad bites were corrected (in cases where it wasn't too late and not too much damage had already been done), many found their headaches and jaw pain disappeared also. They could hardly believe such relief was an unexpected benefit of their orthodontic treatment! But not all changes associated with bad bites are reversible, so it's important to fix them as soon as possible. Abnormal pressure points can wear away tooth enamel and expose the inside part of your teeth (called dentin), causing them to become very sensitive to pressure, heat, and cold. Once this happens, a patient's only recourse is to get a dental crown to cover the exposed dentin. I routinely have parents come in for their kids' treatments and ask for my opinion after pointing out the way their children's lower front teeth have worn down. At this point, the wearing away of the enamel is often too advanced to treat, and I'm not able to offer solutions because the damage is already done.

Bad bites can also lead to gum loss and to bone wearing away from around the teeth. Most of my adult patients, for example, don't lose teeth due to cavities, since most of them have good oral hygiene, but because of bite issues. Their poor bites can cause the supporting bone around their teeth to shrink, leading to periodontal problems and the eventual loss of teeth. Of course, all of these issues take time to develop, and that can be a good thing if it allows time for intervention. But it can also lull people into a false sense of security. Those with bad bites may argue about the need to fix them, saying, "I never got braces, and I'm okay." But just like people with other bad habits (e.g., excessive drinking or smoking) who think they're healthy, those practices usually catch up with them eventually. Problems have a way of getting bigger when they're ignored, and bite problems are no different. Early correction is always the best choice.

6. Isn't there some way to speed up treatment time for my kids? If not, how long does it usually take to have teenagers' teeth straightened?

Orthodontic treatment typically takes one to two years. Metal braces used to be faster than other types, but that's not true anymore. Thanks to new advances in orthodontic technology, clear braces, and even Invisalign, take about the same amount of time to correct your bite. Of course, treatment time also depends on the complexity of your individual case. And since every person's mouth is unique and different, fixing each person's teeth and bite will be different too. Simpler adjustments can be done relatively quickly, while those that are more complex will require comprehensive treatment that takes more time. In these more complex cases, for example, I may need to bring down a stuck or impacted tooth before I can even begin the straightening process. I may also need to align a person's jaw, widen the upper jaw, or advance the lower jaw (when a lower jaw is too small) before correcting the placement of their teeth with braces. This preliminary phase can last about one year or so. Ideally, this phase-one treatment is performed at an early age, when a child is around eight or nine years old. But once a patient is ready for braces, I'm able to reduce the length of their treatment with special techniques such as SureSmile, using computer-guided robotic technologies. AcceleDent and Propel VPro5 are two other accelerative devices I use to decrease Invisalign treatment time.

7. Can you explain in detail how braces are put on teeth? I just want to know what to expect. Is it done during a single appointment, or does it take several? Is it a painful process?

If you were one of my patients coming in to get your braces, I'd place them on your teeth during a single appointment, using a five-step procedure that's quick and painless. First, your teeth will be lightly cleaned to make sure the surface of each tooth is free of any plaque. (This light cleaning is different from the more thorough cleaning and scaling done by a dental hygienist during your twice-a-year visits to your dentist, and it doesn't replace them.) Second, a simple frame-type dental guard is temporarily placed in your mouth to keep the inside of your cheeks away from your teeth, along with a suction tube that removes saliva to keep your mouth dry. Third, an acidic etching solution, or etchant, is applied to your teeth to clean debris off your tooth enamel and prepare the enamel's surface for a bonding agent. Fourth, a primer bonding agent is applied. During the fifth and final step, the actual braces are bonded to each tooth, one by one, and then a special light is used to cure and harden the glue that holds them in place.

> Getting your braces put on is more like having a sticker placed onto each tooth, one at a time.

This procedure isn't painful in any way, and no needle or shaping instruments are used. As a matter of fact, getting your braces put on is more like having a sticker placed onto each tooth, one at a time. Once all the braces are placed, thin wires are attached to the braces using rubber bands. It's a relatively simple process that usually takes only about forty minutes to an hour. Actually, I think most of my patients, especially the kids, find having to sit still without moving—so I can place the braces in the perfect position— is the most difficult part. So it's important for patients to remember to use the bathroom before we start the procedure so it doesn't have to be interrupted.

8. How long do I have to wait to eat after getting braces? Will it hurt when I chew, and do I have to avoid certain foods at first?

After getting braces, you can eat right away. Although your teeth may be tender for several days, eating shouldn't be an issue if you follow a few guidelines. You can expect the tenderness to feel a bit like the muscle soreness you experience after you exercise or work out. That's why I recommend that you stay away from hard, chewy foods during this period, since biting down hard may make your teeth even more sensitive. All things considered, I think it's advisable to stay on a soft diet for the first few days after the braces are placed to allow this tooth sensitivity to pass. But if that warning doesn't deter you from chomping on hard food, you should know eating hard food may cause the slender wires on your braces to bend and pop out of place and start poking you in the cheek. Munching on the wrong food may even cause your brackets (the individual metal pieces attached to your teeth to hold the wires in place) to come unglued from your teeth altogether. So just avoid crunching on hard foods at this time. Although you're allowed to take over-the-counter pain relievers, you need to keep in mind that Advil and Motrin (ibuprofen) can slow down the very tooth movement that's going to straighten your teeth, so it's best to avoid using it once you're wearing braces or clear aligners. To avoid interfering with this essential tooth movement, you can take Tylenol (acetaminophen) instead.

9. What should I do if I need to get braces but I don't have a regular dentist? Don't I need a referral from a dentist to see an orthodontist?

Although family dentists sometimes refer their patients to a particular orthodontist, their referral is simply a recommendation. And the truth is, you don't actually need a dentist's referral to schedule an appointment with an orthodontist in the first place. That said, it's important to maintain good oral health with regular dental visits. Besides, many general dentists know what bite problems to look for during their examinations and will refer patients for braces at the right time—but it doesn't always work out that way. One of my patients, for example, was already fourteen years old when I first saw her and diagnosed her significant jaw issues. Unfortunately, it was several years too late for her to get nonsurgical jaw correction, and her parents were understandably upset. "I don't understand why our family dentist didn't refer us to you sooner," they told me. Although I can't answer that question, I *can* tell you most general dentists just focus on checking for cavities and gum issues and tend to miss bite problems. So it's critically important to be proactive and seek an orthodontist's opinion about the alignment of your child's jaw when they are seven or eight years old. I'm not recommending they start treatment at that age, but it's important that an orthodontist periodically track your child's jaw development so any needed treatment can begin at the right time.

10. After seeing three orthodontists for a free consultation, each prescribed a different treatment approach to straighten my teeth. How do I know which practitioner or recommendation is best?

It's not unusual to get differing treatment recommendations from different orthodontists—each advising you on the best way (in their opinion) to straighten your teeth. That's bound to happen because there are so many diverse orthodontic treatment paths and options available now. Of course, having more choices is a good thing because your treatment shouldn't be a one-size-fits-all solution. I help my own patients decide between braces and Invisalign, for example, and from a variety of different bracket systems and appliances. Like other practitioners, I have my own preferred orthodontic philosophy and approaches. Some prefer removing teeth, and others prefer not to, which is fine. But when seeking an orthodontist's opinion, it's important to ask about the length of their experience and how many similar cases they've treated. Also, keep in mind that different treatment approaches will produce different results—that some approaches may be better than others— and that their outcomes may vary.

When choosing a practitioner, you should definitely ask whether they're a specialist in orthodontics or just a general dentist. Of course, asking friends or other people about their treatment results and their experiences with their orthodontists is a good word-of-mouth option. You can also check online reviews and google practitioners to learn about their philosophies and treatment approaches. Just keep in mind that some orthodontists aren't up to date with newer technologies, and that's an important factor to consider, because opting to use one of the more recent treatment innovations may help you avoid dental surgeries and tooth removal. Such innovations may also shorten your treatment time. I use SureSmile or Insignia advanced braces technology, for example, and in my professional opinion, they not only speed treatment considerably but provide even better results than more conventional approaches. But whether you ultimately opt for Invisalign or braces is completely up to you, depending on what you prefer, since both will straighten your teeth.

11. It's embarrassing to ask, but I want to know if it's safe to kiss my girlfriend who has braces too. Can't my own braces get stuck to her braces and wires if I kiss her?

Everyone probably remembers seeing movie scenes depicting the humorous dilemma of two people with braces getting stuck together while kissing. But the chance of this actually happening is slim to none. Although it's a comical situation full of dramatic potential, I'm happy to be the one to tell you—it just won't happen. That's because braces are made up of two parts: the braces themselves, technically known as brackets, and the wires attached to them. And for the braces on two different people to get locked together, a large number of their brackets and wires would have to come loose simultaneously. Not only that, those components would have to meet in a certain way for them to get tangled up and locked together. So this is one issue involving braces you don't need to worry about.

12. When I need to fly, I'm afraid my new braces will set off the metal detectors as I go through security at the airport. Has that actually happened to anyone?

The myth that braces will set off metal detectors at airports or in other buildings is a common concern many of my patients ask me about. I'm happy to reassure them that wearing braces won't trigger any metal detectors. If I haven't already talked about it with a patient, I sometimes bring up the topic as a joke and advise that they "try not to set off any bells and whistles with your braces." But some of my patients think I'm serious and ask, "Wow, you're right! What do I do now? Do I need to get my braces removed before going to the airport?" I quickly reassure them that's not necessary. So unless you have braces that were designed thirty years ago, you don't need to worry. Modern braces are small and made from light metals such as nickel titanium that won't trigger alarm systems. Even jaw expanders, which have more metal than normal braces, don't contain enough to set off alarms when passing through security. As a side note, I also assure my patients that having braces doesn't increase their likelihood of being struck by lightning either!

13. Seeing how the orthodontist was able to change my teeth and give me a different smile was really interesting. Even though I'm only

seventeen, I'm now seriously considering becoming an orthodontist in the future. What would I need to do?

After you finish high school, you'll need to graduate from a four-year college, then take the Dental Admission Test and apply to a dental college. Although it's not the norm, some students who complete the prerequisite courses required for dental school admission don't actually finish all four years at a college before being admitted. But once accepted by a dental school, you can expect to finish four more years of dental education—with the first two years geared to acquiring academic knowledge and the last two years focused on gaining expertise in the clinical practices needed to actually treat patients. During the first two years, you'll be studying textbooks about dentistry and working on mannequins and fake teeth to practice necessary skills. By your third year, you can expect to start seeing and treating patients under the supervision of faculty and teachers. Having to treat actual patients for the first time can be an unnerving transition. But before graduating from dental school as a dentist with a DDS or DMD, all dental school students must complete different phases of a variety of clinical procedures on real patients.

After graduation, aspiring dentists must pass a board exam in the state where they plan to practice. Those who pass can either start working as general dentists or begin their three additional years of training needed for specialties such as orthodontics and oral surgery. Once you've applied for a specialty residency and have been accepted, you'll need to successfully complete your three years of training in orthodontics. After this three-year residency, you will finally be certified as an orthodontist. As you can see, it's a rigorous course of study but well worth every moment for those who feel called to the challenge!

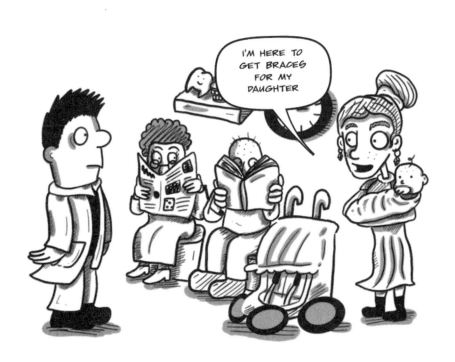

CHAPTER 2

PRETEEN PHASE-ONE EARLY TREATMENT

T he caring parents who come in to my orthodontic office are always eager to find out how braces can help correct their children's misaligned, crooked, crowded, or gapped teeth. Whether their kids are in the second grade or sixth makes no difference—the love and concern of the parents who consult with me is evident in every one of their questions. As an orthodontist who is a parent myself, I understand their worries about how the present and future treatments they choose will affect their children long term. So I want to provide comprehensive answers to the most important questions parents ask as I explain how braces can be crucial for the kids who really require them. I'm always eager to supply the essential information parents need to know about how and *when* to proceed with treatment—knowledge that equips them to make the very best treatment decisions for their children during their critical preteen years.

14. Our orthodontist says my nine-year-old daughter needs to be older before she gets braces, but most of her friends already have theirs. Why do some children get braces earlier? She's complaining about having to wait, and we're wondering why we can't get her braces now. Do we really have to postpone treatment?

Since children mature at different rates, orthodontic treatments must be tailored to each child's unique growth and development pattern. Some kids simply grow faster and are more physically mature than other children their same age. I see children, for example, who have already lost all their baby teeth by the time they're nine years old, while other kids still retain some of their baby teeth when they're fourteen. Personally, I believe straightening teeth with braces should wait until a child has lost most of their baby teeth, which typically happens when they're around eleven or twelve years old. But if a child has jaw problems that need to be corrected, earlier intervention is important. Being fitted with a simple jaw expander appliance to widen their jaw—or to fix an underbite issue caused by a difference in the size of their upper and lower jaws—is often all that's needed. So although I treat many children when they're eight or nine years old to resolve jaw problems, such treatment hardly ever involves straightening their teeth with braces. From time to time, however, I have placed braces on the front teeth of a child as young as eight years old if they were being routinely ridiculed for having crooked teeth. In my professional opinion, it's better to address such social issues by correcting and straightening the child's teeth rather than subjecting them to the mockery of their peers for the next four or five years, during what is a very formative time.

15. When is the best time to get my son braces? Should I wait to see an orthodontist until he's lost all of his baby teeth and his permanent teeth have already come in?

I don't think it's wise to wait that long to see an orthodontist, and I'll tell you why. Children start losing their primary (baby) teeth when they're about six years old, and they don't lose the last of them until they're around twelve. This is the reason I recommend having your child's teeth and bite evaluated when they're seven or eight years of age. It's a good time to check for any early jaw issues and to establish a baseline, so developmental changes in their jaw can be noted and tracked over time. This doesn't mean your child will start treatment then, and they might not need future treatment at all. But it's a good idea to keep track of what's happening as their jaw and teeth are rapidly growing and changing, because that's often the best time to correct problems the most easily.

In fact, for many of the typical jaw issues kids have, the timing of early detection and correction is critical. I've had parents wait until their kids were twelve to bring them in for their first evaluation, only to find out their children had severe bite issues I could no longer correct without surgery. All too often, parents tell me their family dentist told them to wait to see an orthodontist until all of their children's primary teeth were out. But that's a fallacy,

> For many of the typical jaw issues kids have, the timing of early detection and correction is critical.

since I've seen children come in with impacted teeth, too small a bite, an overbite, or an underbite that could have been reversed with early nonsurgical orthodontic treatment. When a child's bite is too small,

25

for example, I can create extra jaw space—even before their baby teeth fall out—with a simple expander that enlarges and maintains the space until their permanent teeth have come in.

This is the reason I advise parents to bring their kids in to see me once or twice a year after their sixth birthday. By monitoring and observing their early development, I'm better able to identify and correct any jaw issues. That way, I'm ready to start the braces process at the most optimal time for them. Some parents are concerned about having to pay for early observational visits, but we don't charge for those appointments, so it just makes good sense for parents to take advantage of these early evaluations and the peace of mind they provide.

16. I have a ten-year-old daughter who recently went to see an orthodontist for an exam and x-ray. The orthodontist advised us to have a few of her baby teeth removed. Since baby teeth will naturally fall out, why do these need to be taken out at all? Wouldn't her baby teeth naturally fall out on their own?

Baby teeth do usually fall out naturally when they're being pushed out of the way by the emergence of a child's permanent teeth. But it's also true that proactively removing baby teeth before they fall out naturally sometimes helps permanent teeth erupt properly—when they couldn't otherwise. Let me explain. A child's baby tooth typically acts like a railroad track that helps guide the permanent tooth into place. But if a baby tooth remains after the roots of permanent teeth have already matured, the baby tooth can actually block the emergence of your child's permanent teeth and prevent them from coming in normally.

This is the reason some children's permanent teeth emerge at the wrong angle (called an ectopic eruption), and they can damage neighboring permanent teeth already in place. A permanent tooth may also get stuck, requiring a minor surgery to help bring it down into its proper position. It's also possible for the roots of a baby tooth to dissolve unevenly and remain after the tooth itself falls out, leaving part of their roots embedded within the bone. Since these residual roots can interfere with the emergence of the permanent tooth trying to take its place, it's better to identify the problem before the roots become too fragile.

An early evaluation and x-ray can prevent this kind of situation by revealing when it's advisable to remove problematic baby teeth so that permanent teeth can erupt properly. But you don't have to worry about early removal of such teeth, even when an orthodontist advises it's necessary for your child. Removing their baby teeth shouldn't pose any problems or have any negative consequences for them. That said, it may comfort you to remember that baby teeth will need to come out eventually, whether that happens with an orthodontist's assistance or naturally.

17. What should I do when my son is still sucking his thumb as an eight-year-old? We've tried everything to break the habit, but nothing seems to work. Can you suggest something to help him stop? I'm worried it will make his teeth crooked. Is that true?

Your child's thumb-sucking habit definitely needs to be corrected as soon as possible. The consequences of thumb-sucking—especially when it is unchecked, continuous, or severe—can lead to serious teeth and jaw problems as your child grows, producing negative consequences for years to come. It can lead to an abnormal open bite, for example, characterized by an oval-shaped gap between their top and bottom front teeth when they smile. Persistent thumb-sucking also causes overjet or buckteeth, marked by front teeth that protrude outward more than the lower teeth. Not only that, this habit tends to constrict your child's upper jaw, making it narrower and almost *V* shaped. It affects the development of their lower jaw as well, causing it to grow downward and back. As if all that weren't bad enough, thumb-sucking can also lead to a tongue-thrusting habit, where a child constantly keeps their tongue postured forward, making normal speech and swallowing more difficult.

Since you're well aware of your son's thumb-sucking problem, it's important to have an orthodontist give him a complete evaluation and diagnosis before seeking treatment options. There may be a number of hidden reasons for his habit, such as breathing issues caused by a narrow upper airway or by enlarged tonsils or adenoids. If this is the case, your child might be sucking their thumb (especially at night) to prop their jaw open so they can breathe better. Although an expander may help improve their breathing, arranging a consultation with an ear, nose, and throat doctor to check for adenoid or tonsil issues would also be wise. But if your child's thumb-sucking habit isn't associated with any airway issues, a simple device called a tongue crib can be used to help him stop. This device prevents a child from putting their thumb or finger between their front teeth and, at the same time, trains their tongue to stop pushing on their front teeth when swallowing.

18. Some of my child's eight-year-old friends already have expanders, but I have no idea how they work. What are they, and why are they needed? Will getting or wearing an expander hurt?

An expander is a simple nonsurgical device that's typically placed in the palate, or roof, of a child's mouth to widen their upper jaw. This is an ideal phase-one orthodontic treatment that's best used when a child still has some of their baby teeth. Using an expander takes advantage of children's natural growth processes to create more space in their mouth before the two halves of the growth plate in their upper jaw fuse after puberty. Expanders are custom made for each individual child and are painlessly placed by fitting them over their upper back teeth. Sometimes referred to as a rapid palatal expander, the lightweight frame of the device works by exerting a gentle pressure that gradually creates more space for a child's crowded or impacted teeth. This widening process can minimize, or even prevent, the need for your child to have tooth extractions later and can actually improve the appearance of their smile.

Another important benefit is the way an expander can easily correct kids' crossbites—a bite problem where the upper jaw is narrower than the lower jaw. This simple bite correction prevents a child's jaw from developing asymmetrically and reduces the potential for adult jaw issues that can be fixed later only with jaw surgery. What's more, I've found that expander therapy can even improve the function of children's upper airways and their ability to breathe. I have successfully treated kids whose mouth breathing was so severe, they couldn't inhale through their noses at all when they first came to see me. Just wearing expanders (for less than a year) enabled them to breathe much more normally. And being able to breathe through their nose is really important for your child's long-term dental health, because beyond issues of comfort, it's essential for the prevention of cavities. Mouth breathing creates a dry oral environment where decay-causing mouth bacteria can thrive in greater numbers.

I'm pleased such huge benefits can be achieved with a device that's so simple and easy to use. Seated in the roof of a child's mouth, an expander is made of two lightweight sections connected with a tiny center key, or screw, which is turned once daily over the course of a few weeks. As the key is turned, the expander gently pushes on both sides of a child's palate to slowly widen it. The expander can either be permanent (fixed) or removable, but in most cases, a fixed expander works best because it requires the least amount of patient compliance, which is an important consideration when treating children. Both types are left in a child's mouth for the same number of months, and using a permanent expander doesn't mean it stays in a child's mouth permanently—the term just refers to the fixed, or more secure, way the expander is placed.

Whichever type you choose for your child, wearing an expander shouldn't ever hurt. Initially, it tends to feel big and odd to kids' tongues—and swallowing and speaking may feel strange to them at first—but only for seven to fourteen days. During that period, you may notice a slight slurring of your child's speech, particularly with words beginning or ending with the letter *S*, but this is typical. If you have them practice reading out loud, most kids will be speaking perfectly normally by the time I check them two weeks later. Although the expander is usually turned (tightened) for only a few weeks, it's left in a child's mouth for an additional six to eight months to make sure the expansion is stable and the bone in their jaw has stabilized. When the expander key is being turned, you may sometimes see a space opening between your child's front teeth, but don't panic; this is normal. The space will gradually close as the teeth drift back together over the course of their treatment.

---

19. A dentist just told me my seven-year-old son's upper front teeth are sticking out because his lower jaw is positioned too far back, and he'll eventually need jaw surgery to fix it. Is there anything else we can do?

If a child's lower jaw is too small, it's very important to begin fixing the problem with a nonsurgical approach when they're around eight or nine years old. That way, they won't have to go through jaw surgery to modify their jaw when they're older. Fortunately, your son is the right age to start this kind of nonsurgical treatment, which can correct his jaw issue in as little as twelve months. In my own orthodontic practice, for example, I frequently prescribe the placement of a fixed Herbst device that a child will wear for about a year as part of their phase-one early treatment plan. This device exerts gentle pressure that increases the size of a child's lower jaw by bringing it forward, allowing the jaw joint to reform in a normal position. Similar removable-type devices such as the Twin Blocks appliance work in a similar way to correct a child's lower jaw when it's not big enough. But starting this treatment early is essential, because after a certain point in a child's development, jaw surgery will be the only way to fix it.

Since identifying this kind of jaw problem early is key to fixing it without surgery, it's important that parents know which outward signs in a child's appearance may indicate they have this issue. An *overjet* (which most people refer to as an *overbite*) is one such indicator. When a child has an overjet, parents may notice their front teeth sticking out, but the appearance of those protruding teeth can be misleading, since an overjet is often caused by a lower jaw that's simply too small. In such cases, the child's upper teeth are actually positioned properly in relation to the rest of their face. Instead, it's the child's lower jaw that's really causing the problem—as well as the big space between their upper and lower teeth—requiring correction.

20. Are underbites genetic? Is there anything I can do to keep one from getting worse? My seven-year-old daughter seems to have an underbite like me, and I'm worried she's going to have a jutting chin that sticks out and jaw pain like I do. Will braces help, or will she need jaw surgery to fix this?

What you call an *underbite* is something orthodontists refer to as a CL3 bite, and it is (unfortunately) true that it's often caused by genetic factors. So the fact that you have one yourself definitely indicates your child's bite should be checked for the problem. In fact, almost 100 percent of the time, an underbite is inherited from one or both parents (or someone else in the family, like grandparents), so your child is obviously more likely to have one too. In such cases, a child should be assessed as soon as possible so they can reap the full benefit of early phase-one intervention treatment if it's needed. This orthodontic evaluation is critically important because parents may not be able to detect an underbite by themselves.

In fact, parents of many of the seven- and eight-year-olds I examine are often surprised when their children's x-rays and measurements show they may be developing underbites—because they haven't noticed any outward signs of their kids' underbites themselves. And that's totally understandable, because the jaw problems preceding the development of an underbite in a growing child can be very subtle.

A child's body will try to compensate for any structural deficiencies in their jaw by changing the way their front teeth meet together, and this unconscious adaptation can effectively hide the problem until it becomes fairly pronounced. This is why it's so important for parents to bring their children in to be evaluated early. If they wait until they see their kids developing an underbite at age twelve or thirteen, it's already too late for nonsurgical correction. That's really unfortunate, because their child has a problem I could have easily prevented without surgery if they had come to see me five years before.

Something many parents don't realize is that some underbites aren't caused by a lower jaw being too big but by their child's upper jaw being too small, from front to back—both widthwise and lengthwise. If caught early, I can correct that with two simple devices: an expander and a face mask. By placing an expander in the roof of a child's mouth, the two halves of their upper arch (palate) can be gently widened over time. And by using a face mask device (also called a reverse pull header) at the same time, I'm able to gradually bring their upper jaw forward. Some kids worry about looking strange wearing the face mask, but they don't need to, because it doesn't have to be worn at school or outside the home. And given the choice, most parents and kids would agree it is far better to avoid jaw surgery by solving an underbite problem with simple orthodontic devices like an expander and face mask. That's why it's so vital that parents bring their children in to be checked when they're seven or eight years old, before the suture joining the two halves of their palate has fused during puberty. In fact, my oldest daughter had an underbite I successfully treated with a face mask and an expander, and it drastically improved the development of her upper jaw. Had I not done anything about it when she was young, she would have needed to have jaw surgery later to fix it.

21. Can I stay with my daughter during her orthodontic visits, since I already do that when she goes to the dentist? Do you ever need to use antianxiety medication when you treat kids the way some dentists do for dental procedures?

In most orthodontic practices, including mine, parents are welcome to come in and observe while evaluations or treatment is given. During my twenty years in practice, I've always done it that way because it's the approach that's most reassuring to both children and parents. I have treated thousands of children, and because some of the kids were very nervous when they first came in, I quickly discovered that it's essential to establish a good relationship with the kids and earn their trust before actually starting their treatment. To accomplish that, I avoid doing active work during the first few appointments. I perform simple but needed examinations instead and use the time to get to know a child and establish open communication with them. Since children need to understand that whatever we do during typical orthodontic visits will not cause them any discomfort, I take the time to assure them of that fact. My staff and I carefully explain how we're going to make their teeth work better, while reassuring kids that we don't need to use any sharp instruments to do that. This approach is so effective, almost 100 percent of the kids I've treated haven't needed antianxiety medication or nitrous oxide (sleeping gas) for routine orthodontic procedures. For exceptionally anxious kids, I've found patience is key to comforting their fears, so I will take as long as they need to feel secure during each appointment. Typical orthodontic treatment is a long procedure—like, say, a two-year process—so there's no need to rush and try to get everything done more quickly than necessary. I've found that slowing down, helping kids feel calm, and proving to them that their treatments won't hurt are all that's needed. After a few appointments, kids will know what to expect and feel confident there's nothing to be afraid of when they come in for their orthodontic visits. Many actually look forward to seeing me!

22. Since my child's teeth aren't crooked, why would she need braces? Aren't braces just for people who want straight teeth?

Just looking at your child's teeth from the front, they may appear straight, but their back teeth could be crowded or crooked, and you might not have even noticed. Yet it's important to detect tooth position problems in the back of your child's mouth as soon as possible, because they can cause food impaction and gum disease later on. It's also crucial to assess whether your child has one of the seven main bite problems that should be corrected with braces. These include crossbite, underbite, open bite, deep bite, crowding, spacing, and protrusion. Like many other teeth or jaw problems, these conditions are most easily treated if they're identified at the right time during childhood when kids' jaws are still growing. One reason they're often overlooked is that children with bite problems can usually still eat and chew without any issues, thanks to the fact that the human body is surprisingly resilient and adaptive. Another reason they go undetected is that serious bite issues aren't always easy to identify unless a child is evaluated by an orthodontist. But left untreated, bad bites tend

> Teeth may crack, break, decay, or wear down when the body can no longer tolerate the uneven jaw pressure that results from a poor bite.

to cause a variety of gum and teeth problems down the road. Teeth may crack, break, decay, or wear down when the body can no longer tolerate the uneven jaw pressure that results from a poor bite. And aesthetically speaking, abnormal bites often cause children's teeth to become progressively more crooked over time.

23. I've made an appointment for my kids to see an orthodontist, but he wants to have x-rays taken as part of their exam. I'm concerned about exposing my children to radiation, so I'd like to skip the x-rays. Is this kind of imaging really necessary?

The diagnostic x-rays generated during an orthodontic exam produce such a tiny amount of radiation, you don't need to worry about your children's exposure to those minute levels. As a matter of fact, your child will be exposed to more radiation just walking around in the sun on any given day. Such low-level radiation exposure is part of everyday life. And just as sunshine is essential for their health, x-ray imaging is an essential component of your children's orthodontic treatments. The images they provide will reveal the true condition of their teeth and jaw and show what specific treatments are required to improve their bites and align their teeth most effectively. A simple visual examination just isn't sufficient. That's why x-ray imaging is so helpful at the beginning of a child's treatment, and it's often the only one needed.

The amount of radiation emitted by x-rays is measured in very tiny units called *microsieverts*. In the US, all of us absorb about 8 microsieverts per day from typical background radiation. But if you were to fly from New York to San Francisco, you would absorb about 40–60 additional microsieverts of radiation. This is due to high altitude causing the air to be thinner, so that fewer cosmic rays (radiation from space) are deflected. And if you share a bed with someone each night, you can add even more to your daily quota, since human beings themselves actually emit radiation! (You didn't know that, did you?) The US Nuclear Regulatory Commission says that the average person is not harmed by the equivalent of 6,200 microsieverts of radiation they're exposed to annually. Half of that amount actually comes from natural sources and half from manmade sources. To put that in perspective, an orthodontist's traditional 2D panoramic x-ray will emit about 8 microsieverts for each exposure, whereas a 3D cone beam computed tomography x-ray, taken with an i-CAT FLX machine, will give out only 5.3 to 6.8 microsieverts during a typical quick scanning.

So as you can see, the amount of radiation exposure for your child having an x-ray is minimal. However, most orthodontists still take exposure to *any* radiation seriously and limit it in every way possible. At my office, for instance, we perform thorough yearly inspections to make certain all of our equipment is operating properly. And our employees wear x-ray sensor badges to measure the amount of x-rays being emitted around the machines. So you can have confidence that your children will be perfectly safe having x-ray images taken and that the amount of diagnostic information obtained from each x-ray is invaluable in designing the best treatment plan for them.

---

24. My eight-year-old daughter needs a space maintainer, and I was told an impression mold of her teeth has to be made. But she has a strong gag reflex. She's worried she may throw up when the molding

material is in her mouth. She's scared and doesn't want to go to her appointment. What can I do?

Traditionally, an orthodontist makes the impressions for a child's braces by creating a mold of their teeth using a puttylike material that's briefly placed in their mouth. This can be an uncomfortable experience for some people—especially children. They may feel as if they can't breathe, and some kids may even have a panic attack. Not only that, when the putty material touches a child's upper palate, it can trigger a gag reflex that makes them throw up, creating a messy and traumatic situation for them.

Although I still do make traditional putty moldings of teeth when they're needed, I also have an iTero Digital Impression System that uses a scanner to create a detailed digitally perfect 3D model of a child's teeth and gums in two to three minutes. Not only is this process far more comfortable than making the old putty-based impressions, but it's faster and more accurate, creating superior impressions that ensure children will have a better-fitting device. During this newer kind of impression-capturing process, your child can breathe or swallow as they normally would, without worrying about putty triggering their gag reflex. So you should definitely call an orthodontist before your first visit to verify they offer the 3D impression technology, because it can make a world of difference to your child. In fact, I've asked many former patients what they considered to be the most difficult aspect of getting orthodontic treatment. Some of those patients said the putty-impression process was the worst part because they actually threw up at an appointment—an experience that was (understandably) traumatic and embarrassing for them.

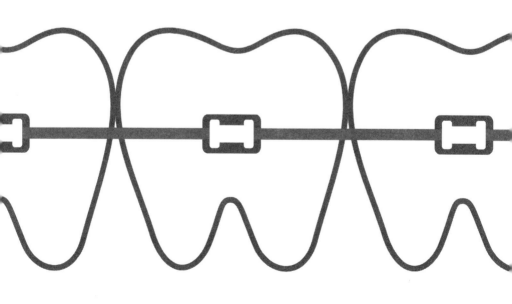

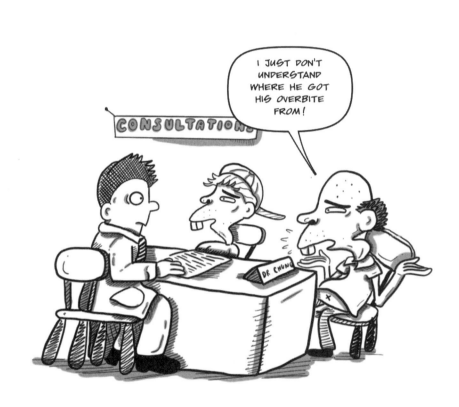

CHAPTER 3

TEEN TREATMENT

When kids become teenagers, I view them as young adults who are mature enough to fully understand the various factors that will affect the success of their orthodontic treatment—as well as the process itself. That's why I work with teens as treatment partners who will be responsible to make key decisions and consistently follow through with the daily steps needed to successfully align and straighten their teeth. My role in that partnership is to share my knowledge and experiences in an individualized way that engages a teen's interest and trust in the orthodontic work I do on their behalf. Their role is to commit to the daily steps needed to complete their treatment plan (with parental support), whether for braces or Invisalign, and to ask questions when they're confused about any of those steps. To help teenagers do that, I've addressed some of the most common questions adolescents and their parents ask when they decide it's time to start fixing their teeth. It's a journey we'll make as a team, working together to prepare them to face their futures with a strong, healthy, beautiful smile.

25. Our dentist says my twelve-year-old daughter is ready for braces, and she's scheduled her for a consultation with an orthodontist. I'm just curious about what will happen during that consultation, and if she's ready, will my daughter get braces the same day? How long will it take to put her braces on? Doesn't it usually take a few hours?

You can expect your daughter's first orthodontic consultation to last about thirty minutes. During her initial appointment, an orthodontist will examine and assess the placement of her teeth and jaw, and if needed, request diagnostic x-ray imaging. Sometimes a second consultation appointment is necessary before a treatment plan can be created to review any complicating factors with a parent. But most times, an orthodontist will present the treatment plan on the same day of the consultation. If it turns out she does need braces and she feels ready, the braces can be put on right away during a process that will take only an additional thirty to sixty minutes. But her teeth will need to be cleaned and prepared beforehand, and careful instructions must be explained so she understands and is reassured about the process.

When Invisalign treatment is chosen instead of braces, your daughter's same-day scanning appointment may be shortened to just ten to twenty minutes, but she will have to wait four to six weeks before her first Invisalign trays are delivered and ready for her to wear. Some offices still create putty molds of kids' teeth for their Invisalign trays, but our office uses digital scanning (no radiation) to determine the shape and position of her teeth. This digital image is sent to Invisalign electronically, but as I mentioned previously, it may take anywhere from four to six weeks to have the actual trays fabricated. Once those are delivered to the office, your daughter will be scheduled for an appointment so the orthodontist can show her how to begin wearing them.

26. After taking my teenage daughter to an orthodontist for an examination and x-rays, he told me one of her canine teeth is stuck high on her upper jaw. I'm upset because he says she needs to see an oral surgeon to try to save the tooth, but she might need an implant if he can't. What do you think I should do?

Upper canines are sometimes called "eye" teeth or "fang" teeth, and because they are one of the last permanent teeth to descend into the mouth, they're also the teeth most likely to get stuck, or impacted. That's because there's simply less room for teeth to erupt in a mouth that's already nearly full of permanent teeth. With that in mind, you actually have two treatment options in a situation like your daughter's where her canine tooth is impacted. The tooth can be removed and later replaced with an implant tooth, as the orthodontist you consulted suggested. Or you can opt to have the tooth moved down with braces. If you choose this second treatment path, an oral surgeon will perform a minor surgical procedure to access the impacted tooth in your daughter's gum. After making a small opening, he'll attach a special bracket and chain (called a gold chain) to the impacted tooth that will gradually bring the tooth down into place. I've successfully done this many times with the help of a 3D cone beam computed tomography scan (CBCT). Although few orthodontists (fewer than 10 percent) have this type of x-ray equipment, the one in our office provides far more accurate and comprehensive 3D views of an impacted tooth than do 2D panoramic x-ray images. In fact, a single 3D scan produces images that can be moved around in a way that shows me not only the exact position of an impacted tooth but also the soft tissues, nerve pathways, and bone around it. That's important because these 3D images allow me to assess how successful this kind of procedure is likely to be for a patient and shows the oral surgeon exactly where to go through the gum to attach the bracket and chain to an impacted canine, so I can begin the braces process. I've done hundreds of cases like this to successfully bring teeth down, and I rarely suggest that a patient have an impacted canine tooth extracted. As a matter of fact, when my own daughter was twelve years old, she had the worst case of impacted upper canines I've seen during my entire career. Most of my colleagues and several oral surgeons told me her tooth needed to be extracted because of its terrible position. (The tooth was high, angled at 180 degrees, and sticking out near her nose!) But I didn't like the idea of extracting it and decided to tackle the problem myself. And the rest is history! She's now a fourteen-year-old with perfect teeth. Because I was able to success-fully resolve such a problematic canine impaction, my colleagues encouraged me to have her case published. I may yet do that, but the point is, I rarely advise removing impacted teeth because it's better, whenever possible, to try to preserve them and bring them down instead.

27. I'm the parent of a thirteen-year-old who will be needing braces soon. But I hated my braces as a kid, and I don't want my son to go through what I did. Are they as miserable as I remember?

Braces have come a long way during the last few decades. As you may remember, they used to be quite big, and their bands or rings sometimes had to be fitted and inserted for each individual tooth. It was like having crowns put on each tooth to create enough pressure to separate the teeth. Nowadays, braces are much smaller, have round edges, and do not go around the whole tooth. And due to improvements in braces technology, small-sized braces can be glued in the center of the teeth instead. We can also use clear ceramic braces instead of the metal kind. Even the metal wires used for braces have changed. Instead of the stiff, stainless-steel wires you probably remember from your childhood, the latest wires are made of heat-activated nickel tantalum that is far more flexible. They produce a much lighter, more gradual force on the teeth as compared to the abrupt force of the old wires. And new innovative technologies such as SureSmile or Insignia can reduce treatment time so much, they often cut the time kids have to wear braces in half. Even more amazing is the fact that it's no longer necessary to get fixed braces on your teeth at all—because you can opt to get clear aligners like Invisalign instead. These are sets of clear plastic trays you can put in and take out of your mouth easily, and you wear a different one every week to move your teeth. So the bottom line is that braces have come a long way! They are much more comfortable, and there are many more options to choose from.

$28.$ Although my fourteen-year-old son had his braces removed six months ago, his teeth have become crooked again. When we went back to see the orthodontist, he told us we'd need to start over with braces. Do you think we made a mistake and got our son's braces put on too early when he was twelve? Should we have waited until he was fourteen or fifteen before starting orthodontic treatment?

It wasn't a mistake to start your son's braces treatment at age twelve, since that's close to the ideal time, when the majority of kids have already lost most of their baby teeth. As to why your son's teeth became crooked again—it probably happened because he wasn't wearing his retainer consistently after his braces treatment ended. Unfortunately, this kind of orthodontic relapse can take a lot of additional treatment time to fix, and it's the reason orthodontists will stress the importance of wearing a retainer in accordance with the schedule they provide. The retainer stabilizes newly positioned teeth and prevents them from reverting back to their original alignment. This is why kids need to wear their retainers all the time (except when brushing or eating) for the first three to six months after their braces are removed. During the next one to three years, they'll need to wear a retainer to bed every night and then wear it two or three times a week thereafter on a permanent basis. Parents will need to monitor their kids to confirm they're wearing their retainers as the doctor ordered, since it's just a fact of life that younger teens may be less responsible and compliant about wearing their retainers consistently. When all else fails, reminding a teen how good their new smile looks may motivate them to keep it that way by using their retainer as directed! Because you asked about the right age for your teen to get braces, I want to caution parents to avoid starting braces treatment too early. If kids still have any of their baby teeth (e.g., before age eleven), they'll have to wait for those to finish falling out while undergoing orthodontic treatment. That means their treatment may take twice as long: three to four years instead of eighteen to twenty-four months. Besides the expense and inconvenience of this longer treatment, wearing braces too long increases the risk of kids getting cavities and stained teeth. Obviously, some eight- to nine-year-old kids need phase-one treatments, but those don't involve putting on braces—phase-one devices (such as expanders and headgear) are used to correct underlying jaw problems. Once a child is eleven or twelve, however, they should be ready for braces treatment, since it's actually best to correct and align teeth before a child's jaw and teeth have fully matured. Aligning teeth gets harder as kids get older, and waiting too long may mean there's more risk to achieving results that are less stable.

29. Do your teen patients ever talk about being made fun of? I'm worried my daughter is going to get bullied for her braces. I know kids get ridiculed for wearing glasses, so won't that happen to kids wearing braces too?

When teens are nervous about getting braces, it's usually because they are worried about how they're going to look. That's why I give them the option of choosing "clear" braces—made of a transparent ceramic instead of metal—because they are far less visible on their teeth than conventional braces. Better yet, I can treat most teenagers with Invisalign now, which is an even more stealth way to straighten their teeth. But believe it or not, I see more and more kids coming in nowadays actually *wanting* to get braces as if it's some sort of rite of passage to maturity. In fact, it's rare to get ridiculed for having braces because so many other kids have them. Most of the kids I see tell me their friends have braces and they actually think it is cool to get them, and they're excited to pick from the variety of different braces colors now available. You would be surprised to see how many parents walk into my office with their teens, because their kids have been bugging them to bring them in to get braces. But this is an age-dependent stage that seems to happen typically between ages eleven and fourteen. By the time those same teens are fifteen years old, most of their friends are done with their braces treatment, and these older kids are suddenly averse to getting them. They're obviously afraid they won't fit in if they're the only ones wearing braces. So it's important to bring your teenagers in to start treatment when they're excited to get braces. At the other end of the enthusiasm spectrum, I see kids who are reluctant to get braces because they're afraid it will be painful. I'm always happy to reassure them that braces aren't like they used to be. These days we have advanced types of braces and wires designed to be gentler and more flexible than ever before. Although some kids experience mild soreness for the first two weeks they have braces, most kids deal with it well and are perfectly fine with wearing their braces after they adjust to them.

30. As a parent, I want all the information I can get about how braces could affect my teen's health. Are there any risk factors to wearing braces? What are the pros and cons? Do the benefits outweigh any potential risks?

The tangible benefits (both physical and emotional) that braces offer your teen far outweigh any potential risks they pose. The most obvious benefit I see is the simple fact that having straight teeth and a better smile leads to higher self-esteem. I've treated quite a few kids who were too shy to smile and unable to socialize because of their crooked teeth. But I saw those same teens transformed into self-assured kids who were able to smile confidently after getting their teeth fixed. Although gratifying, this dramatic outcome isn't all that surprising. Aesthetics is such a huge part of our human interactions; it's literally a life changer. And it is why, later in life, when your teen is a young adult being interviewed for schools and jobs, people will focus on their eyes and smile the most. Even if they're dressed perfectly, but their teeth and smile look unpleasant, the interviewer may evaluate them poorly because of their appearance. Discolored or crooked teeth are frequently (unfairly) associated with a lack of discipline or hygiene, even if that's not the case at all. But beyond the emotional and relational advantages of a better appearance, straight teeth and a correct bite offer many health benefits too. A good bite leads to proper breathing, chewing, and digestion. It can also prevent the development of painful temporomandibular joint (TMJ) dysfunction as well as the grinding and wearing down of a teenager's teeth. And aligned teeth are better protected from the gum disease and halitosis (bad breath) that tend to occur when a teen's teeth are so crooked they can't clean them properly.

> The tangible benefits (both physical and emotional) that braces offer your teen far outweigh any potential risks they pose.

Despite all these benefits, having braces does pose a few risks too—mostly related to potential oral hygiene issues. Having braces makes it more difficult to brush, so if teens won't spend the extra time needed for brushing, there's going to be a potentially higher risk of them getting cavities and stains (white spots) on their teeth. Another far rarer problem with braces is that of root resorption. When this happens, the ends of the roots become slightly blunted as the pressure of braces is applied and the root part of the tooth is moved through the bone. This happens very infrequently, and in most cases, the blunting is minimal and causes few issues. But taking a panoramic x-ray every six months of orthodontic treatment can detect the problem when it occurs and is a good way to check for it so your child's treatment can be adjusted.

31. I know a lot has changed since I had braces as a child, and I'd like to have my daughter benefit from the newest orthodontic treatment available for kids. Which is the one you recommend most highly, and why do you think it's the best?

As with other forms of technology (cell phones, computers, and software), orthodontic technology has improved by leaps and bounds during the last few decades. For starters, we no longer have to take impressions of teeth (moldings) using putty that can cause a gag reflex when it's put in patients' mouths. Instead, we now use digital (radiation-free) scanning of each tooth to create study models and to fabricate appliances, such as expanders, that fit better than ever before. Braces wires have changed too—from the stiff, stainless-steel wires formerly used to tighten traditional braces to softer, more flexible "memory" wires made of nickel titanium. And that's not all. Even the braces themselves have changed, and they're now glued individually to the tops of the teeth, replacing the uncomfortable bands that used to wrap around each tooth. Better still, braces have shrunk in size, and they now come with gates that open and close, allowing the wires to engage more securely, even as they create less friction.

Other innovations include computerized robotic technology such as SureSmile or Insignia that can offer your teen individualized, custom-created braces and wires, allowing accelerated treatment time and more accurate finishes. And improvements in x-ray technology are enabling better orthodontic diagnosis and treatment, thanks to more-detailed 3D images generated with much less radiation. Perhaps best of all, if a self-conscious teen opts not to get braces, they can get clear, invisible treatment to straighten their teeth wearing Invisalign trays instead. Besides their "no-show" appearance, the clear trays are more comfortable to wear, and they make brushing easier for busy teens. Although 20 percent of the kids in my practice opt for Invisalign, it's important to remember that compliance wearing the Invisalign tray is key to success with this approach—so if a teen's not responsible, this might not be the best treatment option for them. Maybe that's why the majority of kids in my practice still get fixed metal braces with SureSmile technology, to get the best possible result in the least amount of time.

32. I'm worried about my son getting cavities and stains while wearing braces. Are there special mouth rinses and other products my son can use to keep his braces clean and strengthen his enamel? Which ones do you recommend? Would he be expected to brush his teeth at school?

I advise teens with braces to use a special toothpaste called Prevident because it has a higher concentration of fluoride to protect their tooth enamel. Since topically applied fluoride has been proven to fight cavities and prevent staining on teeth, I ask all of my patients to switch to Prevident instead of using regular toothpaste. And when they use it, I ask them to spit it out without rinsing their mouth with water or drinking anything afterward for about half an hour. That way, some of the toothpaste will remain on their teeth, giving them a mini-fluoride treatment daily. I also advise them to use a remineralizing toothpaste called MI Paste as part of their daily dental hygiene routine. And if kids have difficulty knowing how thoroughly they need to brush while wearing braces, they can use a toothpaste that tints plaque a blue color, so they can see where they've missed removing it.

Overall, I ask kids to brush well twice a day, once in the morning and once in the evening. But it's really important that they make sure to spend sufficient time (e.g., three to five minutes) each time they do it. The thoroughness of each brushing session is more important than the frequency with which they brush. So it's not necessary for teens to brush their teeth at school. I would rather have kids brush once a day, really thoroughly, than rush to brush five times a day without removing all the plaque that's going to cause cavities. Because it takes twenty-four hours or so for the plaque to develop and lead to decay, it's really important for teens to brush thoroughly enough to remove all the plaque on their teeth at least once daily.

33. Now that my son has braces, we keep having to go back to his orthodontist because they keep coming loose. Is this normal?

Although it may seem like a strange thing for an orthodontist to say, it's actually a good thing for braces to come off from time to time. If too strong a glue is used as a bonding agent, the braces will adhere to the teeth almost permanently. (Think amazing superglue!) Imagine how hard it would be to get those braces off without fracturing tooth enamel when it came time to remove them. Unfortunately, this was a common occurrence when braces glues were first invented, especially when clear braces were being bonded to teeth. Those bonds were so strong that pieces of tooth enamel often broke off when braces were being removed at the end of patients' braces treatments.

So the moral of the story is that braces need to be securely attached without being permanently bonded to your teen's teeth. To ensure that balance, braces should be bonded to healthy enamel. If they're not, and they are bonded at a point where tooth enamel has a defect (indicated by discoloration), the strength of the bond will be weaker than it should be. In addition, braces do not adhere as strongly to the surface of fillings, crowns, or any other dental work using artificial tooth-replacement material. Problems with bonding braces may also occur during the initial bonding appointment if the surface of teeth aren't sufficiently clean and dry. In fact, *any* kind of contamination on a teen's teeth will prevent the braces from adhering well, including saliva. And that can pose a problem for kids who naturally generate excessive saliva. While braces are being bonded to a tooth, any sort of moisture, even a droplet of saliva from a cough, can lead to weaker bonds and overly loose braces.

A teen's eating habits can also lead to braces failure. Chewing sticky food is particularly bad, because it loosens the glue that holds the braces on the teeth. Last but not least, your teen's braces may be coming off due to their biting pattern. Your son may have a deep bite where their upper teeth are constantly hitting their lower braces and causing them to loosen. This is a fairly common occurrence, and when the teens I see lose braces, they usually end up losing the ones from their lower teeth. But having told you all that, I want to reassure you that loose braces are a normal part of having braces, and they don't pose a problem if they're fixed fairly quickly.

34. My teen daughter swallowed one of her brackets today. She's not really concerned and doesn't have any symptoms. What should I do?

If your teen swallows a bracket, don't panic. Most of the time, the bracket will pass harmlessly through their digestive system. Since the bracket is made of nickel and titanium, stomach acid won't completely dissolve it, and you will just have to let it pass through the digestive tract on its own. Ninety-nine percent of the time, that's exactly what happens because the bracket is so small. The only thing a teen and parent really need to watch out for is a bracket going down the windpipe and becoming lodged in a teenager's lung. Having a swallowed bracket end up in a lung is very rare. But in the unlikely event that were to happen, both of you would know right away. Every breath would make a kid wince in pain, and they might feel additional discomfort in their chest, have difficulty breathing, or make a wheezing sound. If a teen experienced any of these symptoms after swallowing a bracket, they would need to get immediate medical attention and have a chest x-ray to make sure the bracket was not in their lung. Fortunately, that scenario is very unusual. As you know, kids eat all kinds of stuff, but you don't worry about it going to their lungs, right?

35. Even though my teenage son is the right age to get braces, he absolutely refuses to get them. He wants Invisalign because it doesn't show. Is Invisalign a good option for kids? Does it work as well as braces?

Most of the time, Invisalign provides the same results braces do and will straighten kids' and adults' teeth just as well. In fact, you'll be happy to know that Invisalign offers an added benefit for kids that braces don't—better oral hygiene. A common problem with braces is that it's not easy for teens to brush or floss around them. And poor dental habits can result in decalcification, or white spots forming on their teeth, along with cavities. So their teeth may end up being perfectly straight but with various stains and marks on them. With Invisalign, this is less likely to happen, because kids get to take the Invisalign trays completely out of their mouths to brush their teeth as they normally would without braces. So in terms of brushing, Invisalign is a much better option for kids.

Another Invisalign benefit is that teens get to eat whatever they want. With braces, they're not allowed to eat anything hard or sticky since their braces and wires might come loose. With Invisalign, this isn't a problem because there aren't any braces to worry about. Another advantage is that when kids play sports wearing Invisalign trays, they're less likely to injure their gums and cheeks than if they had regular metal braces. So why would parents want their kids to have anything but Invisalign? I can answer with one word—compliance. With regular braces, kids comply with the treatment because they have no choice. The braces are literally stuck to their teeth, and they don't come off until their teeth have been moved and their braces treatment ends. But it's not that way with Invisalign. If kids don't wear their clear trays twenty-two hours a day, their teeth won't align as planned, and the results of their treatment may vary. Another problem is that kids can lose their trays. Since the trays are removed when eating and brushing, kids sometimes put them down, forget about them, and leave them behind. So in a nutshell, choosing Invisalign is a great option if your teen is responsible, but it could pose a problem if they're not.

36. Since my son's teeth are very crowded and crooked, there doesn't seem to be enough room in his mouth for all of them. I'm afraid some of his permanent teeth will have to be removed. Is there any way to avoid that?

A few decades ago, the standard approach of many orthodontists was to routinely extract a teen's four premolars during orthodontic treatment. Fortunately, that doesn't happen anymore because the practice resulted in a variety of negative consequences, such as airway problems; sunken cheeks, or a "dished in" face; and narrower arches, which made patients look older. Thanks to advances in braces technology, extracting teeth is now avoided in most cases. Expanders, for example, can be used to create more space for crowded or impacted teeth so they don't have to be removed. And new types of specialty braces, such as Damon Braces, have proven effective in treating tooth-crowding problems without extractions. In my practice, about 90 percent of the children and teens I see complete their orthodontic treatment without needing to have any of their teeth removed. But a few will still benefit from it, and I occasionally recommend it because I practice what I call face-driven orthodontics. That means I strive to create the best possible facial profile for my patients, and tooth extraction can sometimes help achieve that objective. If a teen's front teeth are flaring forward, for example, it can cause their lips to jut out too much. Although this may be fine for a person with lips that don't already protrude, others may want to push their teeth back so the look of their lips creates a more harmonious facial profile they can be proud of.

37. Will getting braces hurt my daughter's ability to play her flute? Can she still play a wind instrument while she's wearing braces?

After getting braces, it typically takes a few days to a few weeks for your mouth and cheeks to get used to wearing them. So in the beginning, playing a wind instrument or singing may feel a little different with braces, and it may take a few weeks to adjust. I once put braces on a twelve-year-old boy whose mom neglected to tell me that he played a musical instrument. Ten days later, I got an angry call from the boy's flute teacher. "Do you know what you've done to Johnny?" he asked heatedly. "I am Johnny's flute teacher, and you have ruined his career! He's one of the top flute players in the tristate area, and now he can't play the flute the way he used to!" He didn't give me a chance to explain the change would only be temporary, and I never heard back from him. But the next time I saw Johnny in my office, I asked his mom if his playing ability had recovered. "Oh, yeah, don't worry about that," she replied. "After two or three weeks, he was able to play perfectly fine." Fortunately, that's typical, but it's always a relief when a musician's abilities are restored—and even improved—after getting braces. That was the case with an opera singer I treated whose singing was initially affected by her braces scraping against the inside of her cheek. But by the time her treatment was finished, she was able to sing more skillfully than she ever had before getting braces, thanks to the improved alignment of her teeth and her corrected bite. She was ecstatic because her front teeth were now placed in a way that allowed a better tongue position that enhanced her vocal abilities.

38. We have an appointment with an orthodontist to get braces for our son, who is active in sports. Will he be able to continue playing football and basketball with braces on? Could this make him more prone to getting injuries?

I advise everyone to wear a mouth guard while playing sports, whether they have braces or not. With that in mind, Invisalign is a particularly good option for kids who are active in sports and need braces. Because Invisalign is a plastic tray that covers the teeth, it can actually act as a small mouth guard that's free of the sharp edges of metal braces. So if your kid is active in sports, you should find out if Invisalign is a good option for them. Unfortunately, injuries while playing sports are relatively common, and having metal braces while participating in different contact sports does increase the *possibility* of getting more soft tissue injuries in the mouth. If a player is hit by a ball on their cheek, for example, the braces may knock against the inside of their cheek, causing irritation and cuts. But braces can actually help protect hard mouth tissues such as teeth and bone. I once treated a girl who slid into second base mouth first while playing softball. This caused two of her front teeth to avulse, or

> Injuries while playing sports are relatively common, and having metal braces while participating in different contact sports does increase the *possibility* of getting more soft tissue injuries in the mouth.

literally crack and fall out of their sockets, due to the force of the impact. As luck would have it, the braces were able to hold those teeth in place and prevented them from falling out of her mouth. Had she not been wearing braces, her teeth would have ended up on the ground. In that scenario, her teeth would have to be retrieved and reinserted, then a dentist would have to apply a splint (essentially a wire) to hold her teeth in place. But because the braces and wires were attached to her teeth and acted as a splint, her front teeth never fell out.

39. Can getting braces negatively affect my fifteen-year-old in any way? Will it keep her from completing schoolwork or cause her to miss school? Since my daughter is an honor student, I'm worried getting braces will hurt her grades. And what about meals and snacks? Can she still eat candy and drink juice?

Fortunately, getting braces shouldn't cause a student to miss school or make completing assignments harder. In fact, braces shouldn't negatively affect their schoolwork in any way. But if they have major exams coming up, you might want to ask your orthodontist to postpone tightening a teen's braces. This will ensure that the minimal soreness that sometimes follows tightening doesn't hamper, even to the slightest degree, your student's ability to take their exams. That's the good news. The bad news is that braces *can* play a disruptive role in a kid's routine school and sports schedules if they insist on eating certain foods that cause braces to break in various ways that require repair. This is why eating any snack or menu item that's sticky or hard should definitely be avoided. If your teen bites down on something hard, for example, it may knock off the bracket holding the wire to a tooth, and it will have to be reglued, which will lengthen treatment time. Or it may bend the wire in such a way that the wire can't do its job properly. I usually give out a list of popular foods to avoid (e.g., chewing gum, hard candies, caramels, popcorn), but it doesn't mention every possible culprit. One time a teen came in with broken braces because he was chewing on ice, and he was upset because it hadn't been on the list of foods to avoid. Another time, a kid was brought in with multiple broken brackets and told me he'd been on a Boy Scout trip and he'd chewed on a tree! So teenagers will definitely need to use their common sense when it comes to snacks if they don't want to spend extra time at their orthodontist's office.

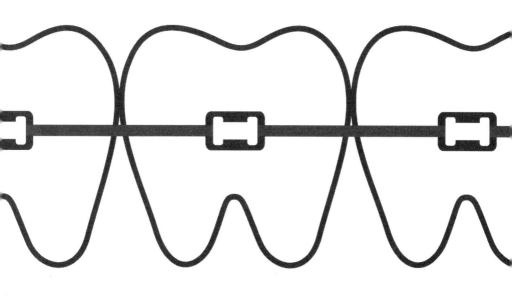

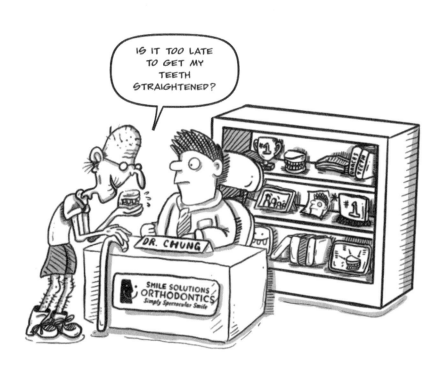

CHAPTER 4

ADULT TREATMENT

Many of my orthodontic patients are adult men and women who never got braces as kids even though they needed them. When they first come in to see me for an evaluation, most are initially insecure about getting treatment because they have so many misconceptions about adult braces. I'm always happy to see the relief on their faces when I tell them that no one is too old for braces, because teeth can be moved at any age. Like my younger patients (and their parents), they ask a lot of insightful questions about getting orthodontic treatment. So I'm sharing some of my answers as a reliable information resource for those of you "big kids" who know knowledge is power. You may have already gotten braces and started treatment or are seeking expert information about their tangible benefits for the future. Either way, the following information will prove very helpful when it comes time to make key decisions about how to best fix your teeth and optimize your smile.

$40.$ Many years ago, my dentist told me I needed braces for my bite issues. I never got treatment back then, but I think I'm finally ready to start braces even though I'm fifty-eight. Am I too old to get them? Is there anything I need to do first?

I'm really happy to tell you it's never too late to get braces, and you're definitely not too old to start treatment. Thanks to all the new innovations in braces technology, now is actually the best time for adults to get them. And it's been very rewarding to see my adult patients' lives so dramatically improved after getting braces. Embarrassed about their crooked teeth, some had become so shy, they were afraid to smile and socialize. But that all changed once their teeth were aligned and their smiles were transformed. Having straight white teeth so boosted their self-confidence, their personalities blossomed in a way that has positively affected every area of their lives, including their marriages, jobs, and social lives.

Some of my adult patients actually cry when their braces come off and they get to see their new appearance for the first time. All of them say they regret not getting treatment earlier, and they wonder why they waited so long to start. For some of these patients, straightening their teeth and widening their upper arch gave them a wider smile and a more youthful look that made them feel younger and more energetic. Of course, there are

> The health of your teeth and gums will allow your natural teeth to last longer, and correcting a poor bite prevents bone loss in your jaw and the further wearing down of your teeth and the deterioration of your gums.

many other benefits to going ahead with adult braces besides aesthetic ones. Beautiful teeth need to be healthy too. The health of your teeth and gums will allow your natural teeth to last longer, and correcting a poor bite prevents bone loss in your jaw and the further wearing down of your teeth and the deterioration of your gums.

So now that you're ready to start treatment, I recommend you see a general dentist first for a regular cleaning and checkup. You may have issues with gum and bone loss I don't usually see in children or young adults. Ask your dentist whether your teeth are in good condition to start orthodontic treatment. It may be necessary to get a few teeth patched or to have some cavities fixed before beginning treatment. And you might need to see a periodontist who specializes in gum issues to check you over too—just in case you have any issues that could affect your braces treatment. Once those precautions have been taken, you're all set. In essence, healthy teeth can be moved at any age, so that means yours can too. I have patients who are currently in their fifties, sixties, and seventies who are undergoing treatment right now or who have already finished their treatment with great success.

41. Is it okay for me to get braces if I'm pregnant? I still want to get my teeth fixed, but would you advise I wait or go ahead with it?

Pregnancy doesn't have to prevent you from getting braces. In fact, I've had many patients who successfully finished their treatment after getting pregnant halfway through it. Still, it's good to keep in mind that most orthodontic treatment isn't started to resolve an urgent medical problem. What I mean is that most orthodontic issues won't have negative, short-term consequences if those issues aren't immediately corrected. Bite and alignment problems *do* need to be fixed, and they will have long-term consequences if they aren't fixed, but correcting them isn't something urgent. I ask my pregnant patients to discuss getting braces with their obstetrician and general dentist before starting treatment because pregnancy may bring about bodily changes that can affect your treatment. During pregnancy, for example, hormonal changes can cause a woman's gums to weaken temporarily, which may make them more vulnerable to gum diseases such as gingivitis or periodontitis. This is also why you'll have to be extra careful with your oral health if you're already undergoing orthodontic treatment during pregnancy. Of course, you shouldn't get x-rays when you're pregnant either, so that poses a problem. Because x-rays must be taken before starting treatment, and sometimes midway through its course, I typically ask my patients to wait until pregnancy is over to get braces. But if one of my patients becomes pregnant after their treatment's already started, I will continue it, but I won't take any x-rays during their pregnancy. I'll also slow down the rate at which I'm moving their teeth, and I ask those patients to see their general dentist more frequently for more detailed checkups and cleanings.

42. Someone just told me I can get my teeth fixed right away with instant orthodontics and veneers without having to wait a year for results like I would with regular braces. Since I have a gap and need to get my teeth straightened, are these good options for me?

I'm glad you asked, because it's important you know that "instant orthodontics" isn't really orthodontics at all. Instead, it's a dental procedure that requires you to have your teeth drilled down so that either porcelain (tooth-colored) crowns or thin veneers can be placed over what remains of your teeth. Cosmetically speaking, this approach is used to change the shape and size of your teeth so they look the way you want. But it does so by irreversibly changing your otherwise healthy teeth. When a tooth needs to be drilled a lot to look a certain way, for example, you may have to get a root canal done. So basically, it's a dental procedure performed to strip down teeth before new crowns are placed over the top of teeth to "instantly fix" them. In my opinion, this is a poor option that can harm your teeth to fulfill a cosmetic objective. And although a few of my patients have benefited from a combination of traditional orthodontics and the use of veneers and crowns, instant orthodontics alone won't give you those benefits. That's because the approach is obviously not the same as orthodontics where your natural teeth are preserved, moved, and aligned to function even better after treatment.

Anyone considering the instant orthodontics approach should remember that a person is asking for trouble whenever they get crowns. That's because crowns will inevitably need to be replaced with new ones when the old crowns start to "leak," a situation that often requires more of the natural tooth to be ground down. Although the expense of creating veneers and crowns for each tooth can be high, their average lifespan is only seven to ten years. If I were you, I wouldn't want to have to keep paying for new crowns, for every single one of my teeth, for the rest of my life. I also wouldn't want to feel a synthetic material on all of my teeth with my tongue. And in cases where spaces are closed by getting new crowns, these "teeth" usually end up looking much bigger than normal (since you are filling in the space by inserting a bigger crown on top of what remains of your natural tooth). The unwanted space between your original teeth may be gone, but your modified new teeth may end up looking bulky and unnatural. So I'm not really surprised when adults come in to see me because they're unhappy with how they look after getting these kinds of crowns done. But once their natural teeth have been cut down to accommodate a crown, it's a choice they obviously can't undo.

Having said that, I *do* think there are specific situations in which veneers or crowns can be a better option than braces. Braces cannot change the *size* of your teeth, but veneers or crowns can. If your front teeth are too small and have a gap between them, for example, it may be preferable for you to increase the size of your teeth by getting veneers, rather than closing the space with braces. And if your teeth are discolored or have an odd shape, crowns or veneers may be your only solution because, unlike braces, they can change the color and shape of your teeth to look the way you want. So if you're someone who needs to alter the size and shape of abnormal-looking teeth, cosmetic dentistry's veneers and crowns may be your best treatment choice.

43. What are lingual braces? I've heard they're impossible to see when someone has them. If that's the case, why wouldn't everyone get them? Are they a good option instead of metal braces? Am I a candidate?

About 20 percent of my patients are adults, and most of them prefer something more aesthetically pleasing than metal braces. If that's the case for you too, lingual braces are a good choice because they're bonded behind your teeth, rather than in front like conventional braces. I have several patients who have lingual braces in my practice, and they like the way they're completely hidden behind their teeth. These are actually the most discreet type of braces available and are even less visible than Invisalign.

Despite this aesthetic advantage, there are some downsides to lingual braces you should consider before selecting them:

- Your tongue may become irritated because it will be constantly touching the metal braces bonded to the back of your teeth.

- Oral hygiene may be an issue too because plaque, or calculus, is more likely to build up behind your teeth where the braces are hidden.

- You may also experience speech issues since the braces will be right next to your tongue, making it difficult to articulate clearly.

- Lingual treatment is more technically sensitive and takes longer to finish properly. It's also important to point out that the final result is usually not as good as it is with metal or ceramic braces that have been bonded to the front of the teeth.

Of these issues, I've found most of my patients with lingual braces have the most difficulty coping with the last two issues.

Although tongue irritation gets better after two or three months of wearing lingual braces, speech issues don't really improve. I've found it's almost impossible for adults to change their speech patterns. So you'll have to be okay with having some pronunciation problems (especially *S* and *T* sounds) if you decide to get lingual braces. Also, from my experience, lingual braces treatment always takes longer and is harder to finish compared to labial braces (those on the front of the teeth). Another factor to keep in mind is that lingual braces are typically much more expensive than the labial type or Invisalign. Other treatment choices include ceramic braces (clear or tooth-colored braces). But the wires of these braces are still metal, not tooth colored, so you'll see a wire going across your teeth. For a lot of my adult patients, however, just having clear braces is enough to make them happy.

44. I'm trying to decide whether to get Invisalign or braces. I don't really prefer either one. What are the pros and cons?

For the majority of my patients, the main benefit of Invisalign is in its aesthetic value. Most people won't even notice they're wearing Invisalign, whereas the fact that you're wearing braces will be obvious every time you smile. Another big advantage of Invisalign is that it's a much more comfortable treatment compared to braces. In fact, there's virtually no discomfort when Invisalign is properly used. That's because braces require more pressure, and there will be more soreness as the braces are gradually tightened over the course of treatment. Brushing and maintaining proper oral hygiene is much easier with Invisalign too, since you can clean your teeth like you normally would. Braces, on the other hand, tend to make brushing a challenge since the brackets and wires attached to your teeth make it more difficult to brush and floss properly. In addition, Invisalign won't limit what you eat like braces do, so you won't have to change your diet. But once you're wearing braces, you won't be allowed to eat anything sticky, hard, or chewy. So it's easy to see Invisalign has a lot of advantages as a treatment option.

There *are* a few downsides, however. One of the biggest problems stems from drinking anything other than water (such as coffee or carbonated drinks) with Invisalign trays in your mouth. That's because sugary liquids get stuck between the tray and your teeth, causing stains, cavities, and other decay problems. So it's critically important for patients to remove the trays while eating and drinking anything (other than water). It's also a problem that the success of a patient's Invisalign treatment depends on how compliant they are wearing the clear trays that are straightening their teeth. They need to be worn full time (at least twenty-two hours a day). I've had some of my adult patients actually come right out and tell me, "I don't want to have to remember to take this thing in and out of my mouth all the time. I know myself too well. It just won't happen. So I want something permanent instead."

And some of my patients like the fact that they can choose from clear braces, and even gold-colored braces, and choose to make a style statement out of wearing them. That's probably just as well, since traditional braces can move their teeth faster and more efficiently than Invisalign. That's especially true when adults have teeth that are so severely crowded, individual teeth will have to be turned and rotated into proper alignment. And among patients who need to have a tooth extracted, braces and wires may be more efficient in closing the space that creates. So making the decision between Invisalign and braces really depends on first figuring out what kind of person you are. If aesthetics, comfort, and convenience are most important to you—and you know you will be responsible wearing your clear Invisalign treatment trays—then I would advise you to go with Invisalign. But before starting treatment, be sure to ask the orthodontist if braces and wires would be better (in terms of result and speed) for your individual teeth and jaw.

45. When I got Invisalign, the orthodontist put a lot of little bumps on my teeth, and I don't like them. I thought Invisalign was supposed

to be totally invisible. Why do I need to have these little nodules stuck to my teeth?

When you get Invisalign, the tiny tooth-colored dots placed on your teeth are called attachments, and they help your Invisalign aligners move your teeth. They're placed strategically on your teeth to shift each individual tooth in a very precise way that's been predetermined by your treatment plan. The attachments are made of composite filling material that's bonded to your teeth, and their shape and type are critical to pushing the teeth where they need to go. They can be circular, square, rectangular, or triangular depending on whether a tooth needs rotation, intrusion, or extrusion. So the type of attachment you receive on each tooth depends on the particular way it needs to be shifted. Since teeth are slippery and the Invisalign trays are plastic, attachments are specifically placed to act like a handle that enables a tray to latch onto your tooth and move it.

When Invisalign first came out more than two decades ago, attachments hadn't been developed yet, and treatment outcomes were limited because they relied on the clear trays alone. Since that time, the company that makes Invisalign has invested a lot of money into researching how to use their clear trays to align teeth most efficiently and effectively. Thanks to the type and shape of the attachments they've developed, their clear trays can now be used to move and straighten teeth in a way that wasn't previously possible with Invisalign. In fact, the technology has improved so much, it now works as well as braces for most people. But I still have some patients who absolutely don't want the attachments, especially on their front teeth, and I sometimes have to remove them. Before doing so, however, I make sure the patient understands their Invisalign treatment will take longer, and the desired result may not be possible without adding braces for a short time at the end of their treatment.

46. I really don't want to get braces, period! I don't even want to have clear braces, but I've heard good things about Invisalign. How would it work if I opted to try it to straighten my teeth?

Invisalign treatment relies on using a series of custom-made clear plastic trays (called aligners) to straighten your teeth over time. Because each tray will shift your teeth slightly, wearing a number of different trays (around thirty) will gradually move your teeth into their correct place. To construct those trays, your teeth must first be digitally scanned to map out their existing positions. If digital scanning isn't available, an orthodontist will make physical impressions of your teeth by having you bite into a puttylike molding material. Since that makes some patients uncomfortable—mainly because it can trigger their gag reflex—I prefer to use radiation-free digital scanning in my practice. Those scans are uploaded into software called ClinCheck to digitally predict the way your teeth will need to move over the course of your treatment. Using this information, I create a detailed treatment plan that maps out the direction each tooth needs to shift to achieve its final position in your upper or lower jaw. After electronically communicating that plan to Invisalign, the company will make a series of trays that reflects the incremental changes needed to straighten your teeth. Once these are sent back to me, I'll meet with you to show you how to use the aligner trays you'll need to wear full time, twenty-two hours a day (except when eating and brushing), until your treatment's complete.

47. As a twenty-eight-year-old guy, I'm embarrassed to admit dental procedures make me nervous, but I really need to get my teeth fixed. My wife makes fun of me because I'm afraid to get braces if it means I'll have to deal with needles and shots as part of the treatment. Are there any braces I could get that don't cause any sort of pain?

I have good news for you! You can stop worrying that getting braces is a painful procedure and go ahead and have your teeth straightened. I can assure you that the actual procedure is not painful and that no shots or needles will ever be used during orthodontic treatment. As a matter of fact, sitting in a dental chair while being fitted with braces can actually be a relaxing experience! After the procedure is done, most people are so pleasantly surprised they ask me, "Is that it?" They're obviously quite relieved they didn't have to endure some level of discomfort. Just to make sure it stays that way, I provide treatment modalities such as AcceleDent SoftPulse Technology to speed up overall treatment time and minimize any residual pain or discomfort from being fitted with braces. I also offer TruDenta therapy and cold laser therapy to relieve tight muscles and tone down nerves with the potential to trigger dental pain. In other words, getting braces should never be a painful process.

That said, people *do* have different degrees of pain tolerance, and I've seen adult patients who

> You can stop worrying that getting braces is a painful procedure and go ahead and have your teeth straightened. I can assure you that the actual procedure is not painful and that no shots or needles will ever be used during orthodontic treatment.

are so sensitive, they can't even tolerate the simple scaling a dental hygienist uses to clean their teeth. But for most people, having braces put on won't be painful at all. And even if you're like my more sensitive patients, you're only going to feel a slight soreness for two or three days after you first get braces—or after each of your adjustment appointments (usually every six to eight weeks) when your braces are tightened. This soreness is similar to the minor muscle ache you might feel the morning after working out. Still, if you want to straighten your teeth with the least amount of discomfort, you could choose Invisalign treatment (clear aligner trays), which is typically more comfortable than metal braces. Wearing Invisalign aligners does require more self-discipline than braces, however, because they must be taken out of and put back in your mouth every time you eat or drink anything except water.

48. After a consultation with one orthodontist, I was told my case is too complex and that he wouldn't feel comfortable treating me with Invisalign. I went for a second opinion and was told that I'm definitely a candidate for Invisalign. What gives? How do I know which of them is right?

Speaking from experience, I would say *both* of them are right! Whether an orthodontist recommends Invisalign as an alternative to braces really depends on an orthodontist's level of expertise providing that particular treatment. And that comes, quite frankly, with experience. There are patients I never would have treated with Invisalign a few years back that I'm now treating successfully and confidently. So the first orthodontist you consulted might have simply felt more comfortable doing braces instead of Invisalign, due to his lack of experience with that treatment option. Now that I've personally used Invisalign to treat hundreds of patients over the last twenty years, I can highly recommend it. In fact, the improvements in Invisalign technology have been so significant, I can now treat virtually every one of my patients with Invisalign and get the same, or even better, results than I do using traditional braces. It wasn't always like that though.

I won a raffle at a convention back in 1998 for a free Invisalign case (meaning Invisalign would let me treat one patient without any lab fee). Back then, Invisalign was such a new technology I wasn't even sure I could use it effectively, so I didn't use the prize for the next three years. Then in 2001, I had a patient come in who was adamant about not wanting braces, because she wanted something more aesthetic instead. Although she wasn't asking for Invisalign specifically—because nobody really knew about it back then—I remembered the raffle prize I'd won and decided to offer her Invisalign treatment at a huge discount. Since it was my first time using the treatment, it was a struggle, and I didn't quite get the result I wanted. So I eventually had to put braces on her to finish aligning her teeth.

That less-than-perfect outcome was the result of the fact that Invisalign technology was still in its infancy, and I wasn't yet proficient using it. But as I started doing more and more Invisalign treatments, and the technology itself advanced, I became comfortable providing the treatment and gained the experience and proficiency I have today. So even though I'm sure you're a candidate for Invisalign, I often find a hybrid combination of Invisalign and braces treatment is the best approach for more complex cases. In fact, some corrections are best done by starting out with braces for two or three months, then switching over to Invisalign for the remaining fifteen months of treatment.

$49.$ My job requires me to talk constantly. Will it be harder to speak clearly once I have braces on? Will my speech be affected in any way?

Since normal braces are placed on the outside (front surfaces) of your teeth, having them shouldn't affect your speech at all. During all my years of practicing orthodontics, I've not had a single patient come back to me complaining that their speech had been affected in some way. That makes sense, since traditional braces are kept well away from the tongue. The same can't be said for lingual braces, however, because these braces are placed on the back of teeth where they *will* make contact with the tongue. As a result, lingual braces have the potential to cause rather significant speech issues. Invisalign can also cause speech changes in some patients because the plastic trays cover the back of the teeth, but it's to a much lesser extent than with lingual braces. The reason Invisalign trays affect speech is that even though the trays are thin, when a person's tongue touches their teeth to make sounds, their tongue will hit the tray, resulting in slight differences in pronunciation. Fortunately, almost 99 percent of my patients who undergo Invisalign treatment do not complain about speech changes while wearing their trays. But if you're still concerned about the possibility, you can remove the Invisalign tray to talk whenever you need or want to.

$50.$ Since I'm a professional singer, I'm worried about braces ruining my career. Will braces affect my singing?

Although you may experience some alteration in your singing while wearing braces, the end result of your treatment should actually improve your singing ability—once your teeth and bite have been corrected. That was certainly the case with a professional opera singer I treated who was very concerned about braces being detrimental to her voice. After I first put her braces on, she complained about the negative effect to her singing as her mouth and tongue adjusted to the feel of wearing her braces. This was especially difficult in her case, since she had to move her mouth when it was wide open to sing, and the inside of her lips would touch the brackets and cause some irritation. But over time, this irritation completely disappeared as her teeth became aligned properly and her front teeth were moved into a better position. In the end, she was happy to report that she was able to make certain vocal sounds far better than she had before she'd gotten braces. An additional benefit of her treatment was that her temporomandibular joint (TMJ) issues improved over time. Having to keep her mouth open very wide while singing opera had put so much stress on her jaw joint that she'd routinely experienced pain and clicking sounds in her TMJ during and after rehearsals and per-formances. Although those TMJ symptoms did not go away com-pletely, they improved considerably after her bite was corrected.

$51.$ Because I have a dental phobia, I'm scared of needles. Will you be using needles if I come in to get braces? And do you need to take impressions of my teeth? I once threw up in the middle of that process, and I gag when I have to bite into dental film. Can I avoid any of this?

I want to assure you that no sharp instrument like needles will be used for routine orthodontic procedures such as placing or removing braces. You will always be in control of what procedures you choose to undergo, and painless procedures have become standard. As for making impressions or molds of your teeth, I occasionally still ask for those in some cases, but you can choose to have iTero digital scanning instead. In my office, this kind of scanning allows me to get more accurate models of your teeth (with no radiation) by briefly sweeping a special wand over your teeth for three to five minutes. A lot of my patients appreciate this option since, like most people, they obviously don't enjoy the experience of gagging and throwing up. And you don't have to worry about having to bite into film cards while getting an x-ray, since most orthodontic offices don't use that kind of x-ray anyway. Instead, you'll typically be asked to stand still for about twenty seconds while a panoramic or cephalometric x-ray is taken.

52. Even though I had braces when I was young, I can see my lower teeth shifting and getting crooked again. My upper teeth are still pretty straight. So can I just get braces for the bottom ones?

The short answer is yes, you can just get braces for your bottom teeth. But I wouldn't recommend it. Think of teeth in the mouth as a gear system in which the top and bottom teeth must mesh together correctly to exert the force needed to chew food. Like intersecting puzzle pieces, or fitting the right size lid to the mouth of a jar, they need to join properly. Just straightening your bottom teeth will change the way your lower and upper teeth interact, and it may create bite issues that lead to wear facets. So when one of my patients comes in thinking they just want lower braces, I explain that giving them lower braces will certainly straighten their lower teeth. But that change may actually give them a worse bite than they started out with, and it could do the same to you. It's a big problem—called malocclusion—when newly straightened lower teeth no longer fit

79

your upper teeth. Your upper and lower teeth may even look straight, but if they don't meet properly, your teeth simply won't be able to do the job they're designed to do. So it's critical that I don't simply patch up cosmetic issues. Many times, it's actually better to leave crooked upper or lower teeth alone than to implement a partial fix that may create more problems. Does that mean I never treat only partial teeth? No, it doesn't. I *do* sometimes put braces on a patient's lower or upper teeth alone, but only after creating and evaluating diagnostic images to make sure such treatment won't cause bite problems. I'll always discuss all possible treatment options, but it's only logical that limited treatment will also limit a patient's expected outcome.

53. Would it be okay to have my family dentist fit me with braces, since he says he can do it? Can I get the same result if he does my orthodontic work, or do I need to see an orthodontist? What's the difference between a dentist and an orthodontist anyway?

Although many general dentists can, and do, perform orthodontic work, this is a fairly recent phenomenon. So you can certainly have your dentist do your braces if you like, but your treatment experiences and outcomes will be somewhat different than if you use an orthodontic specialist. Orthodontists like myself are specialists for a reason, and we don't practice general dentistry, because braces are all we do. An orthodontist, like me, is a general dentist who has gone to school for an additional three years of training to learn how to best provide orthodontic treatment. Because we orthodontists are more knowledgeable and efficient as specialists who only straighten teeth, it's logical that an orthodontist is better qualified to provide the best treatment approaches and outcomes. It's like that with any medical specialty, whether it's obstetrics, plastic surgery, or any other area of medical expertise. Family medicine doctors might perform such specialty procedures competently, for example, but most people seeking treatment for specific medical problems will prefer specialists because they have the most knowledge and experience to treat a particular malady most effectively. Likewise, as an orthodontic specialist, I can provide more treatment options (not just limited to Invisalign) and use the latest technology to straighten your teeth the most quickly and comfortably. Plus, an orthodontist's fees are usually comparable (or only slightly higher) than those of a general dentist, so it only makes sense to have an orthodontist fix your teeth.

54. Can I still get braces even though I have some crowns, root canals, and fillings? I also have some missing teeth. But I've always wanted to get my teeth straightened. Can you still do it?

I'm glad to assure you that having dental work does not prevent anyone from getting braces! That's because it's perfectly fine to place braces on crowns or teeth with fillings or root canals to straighten them. Typically, braces glues are designed to bond only to natural tooth enamel. However, even in cases where braces have to be bonded to a tooth with a filling or a crown, I can use a special adhesive that allows them to adhere to this kind of dental work. I can also opt to use Invisalign instead of metal braces. And if you have a large filling in a tooth, a form of braces called a band can be wrapped around it so that it surrounds the whole tooth and prevents further cracking of the filling. The only time this method won't work is if the tooth has an existing filling that needs to be repaired or restored by a general dentist, which needs to occur before I can start treatment. And if you are missing some teeth, orthodontic treatment will actually benefit you if you need to alter the size of a gap. I can close the space by moving your teeth together or widen it even more to make room for an implant or bridge, if that's what is needed.

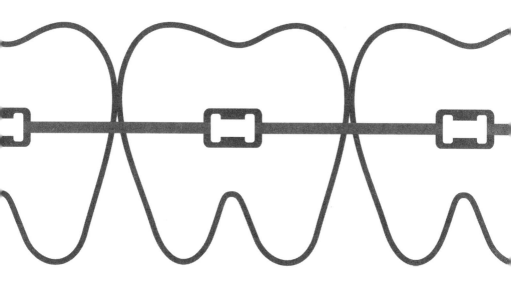

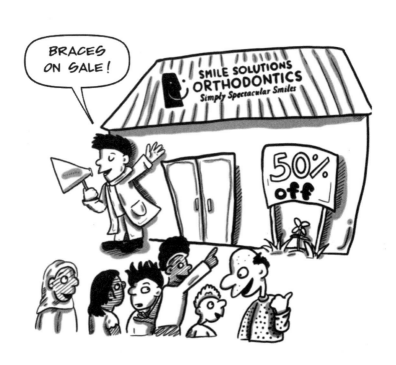

CHAPTER 5

FEES AND INSURANCE

M any who need orthodontic treatment will never come in to see me for a free consult, because they don't think they can afford it for themselves or their kids. That is really unfortunate because they may never find out how surprisingly affordable this kind of treatment really is. And what's worse, they'll never experience the life-changing benefits of a healthy smile that are so accessible with braces or Invisalign. I wish everyone knew that most orthodontists offer initial, no-cost consults and evaluations like I do, and financing options are available to make treatment affordable for just about everybody who needs it. Having your kids come in to see me for a no-cost examination is particularly important since early phase-one orthodontic treatment may be all that's needed to save your child from jaw surgery or lifelong jaw problems that can be readily fixed when they're six to eight years old. So many parents regret it later, especially when they find out they could have easily paid for it. When you consider the cost of an automobile, or even what you'd spend vacationing for a week at a beach house during the summer, getting treatment to fix a bad bite or misaligned teeth is a wise use of your resources. That's why answering your questions about the cost of orthodontics is so important. I never want anyone to sacrifice receiving necessary orthodontic treatment due to cost concerns, so I spread the good news about its affordability as widely as possible.

55. How much will treatment cost? I'd like to get braces, but I'm wondering if I can actually afford them. Can you give me some idea of what people usually pay?

The national average for the cost of orthodontic treatment typically ranges anywhere from $4,200 to $7,600. But you might pay less or more than that depending on your age, your insurance plan, and the kind of treatment approach you need. Different types of treatment include lingual braces (worn behind the teeth), metal braces, clear braces, or the braces-less Invisalign option. After careful evaluation, I'll recommend the type best suited for you, based on the condition of your existing teeth and bite. Of course, some cases are simply more complex than others. And because the position of your teeth and the characteristics of your bite are unique, the solutions used to correct them will be individualized too. More complex cases may require surgery, some teeth removal, the use of additional devices, or longer treatment time. Children's teeth, for example, are often treated in two phases, with early (phase-one) intervention being completed between ages six and nine, because that's the best time to correct a bad bite.

    Although orthodontic insurance will cover some portion of

orthodontic treatment, it's important to make sure you know what fees are included and which are not—because even what's covered will be deducted from the total treatment fee costs. If the total cost of your treatment is $6,000, for example, and insurance covers $2,000 of that, you will still need to pay $4,000 for your portion. Because dental insurance doesn't usually cover the full (if any) costs of getting braces, many orthodontists offer payment plans to make treatment affordable. It's always a good idea to inquire about those plans and to ask your orthodontist about military, professional, sibling, teacher, and paid-in-full discounts or any other type of fee reduction they might offer. Many orthodontists are willing to work with you to make the fee affordable so you can reap the benefits of getting a healthy smile for yourself and your children.

56. What does an orthodontist's fee typically cover? I went in for a free consultation and got an estimate for the cost of my braces treatment. But will the fee I was quoted cover everything from beginning to end?

Your question regarding the total cost of orthodontic treatment is a good one because each orthodontist will charge differently, and it's up to you to ask for a detailed breakdown of their treatment fees. I always welcome and expect such inquiries from my new patients who come in for their no-cost consultations, and you shouldn't be embarrassed to address the topic. The reason it's so important to ask about fees is because some orthodontists' charges are all inclusive, and some are not, so it's

> Each orthodontist will charge differently, and it's up to you to ask for a detailed breakdown of their treatment fees.

always a good idea to ask about any additional costs you might incur. Since the fee varies for each orthodontist and office, you may need to have them spell out exactly what's included in their total fee and what is not. Otherwise, you may unexpectedly end up paying extra for extended treatment time or for specific types of treatment such as clear braces or Invisalign. The Invisalign treatment fees of some orthodontists, for instance, may only include the cost of your first set of aligners, and if any additional treatment (called refinement) is needed, you might be charged extra for that. You may also pay extra for various types of retainers, including the permanent kind—or those you need to wear after your braces come off. You could even be charged for the individual brackets that occasionally break during the course of your treatment. With all that in mind, don't forget to ask about the benefits, availability, and costs of additional supplemental devices such as AcceleDent, VPro5, SureSmile, Insignia, TAD mini-screws, and laser therapy since these can facilitate the speed and success of your treatment so tremendously. Like any other consumer purchase, it's wise to weigh the pros and cons of each treatment and decide which treatment provider can offer you the most for your money.

57. I have three children who need braces, and I want them for myself too. But I'm not sure if I can afford it. Will my dental insurance cover the cost of orthodontic treatment, or should I try to sign up for an additional insurance policy to cover it?

Many people who have dental insurance assume it covers orthodontic treatment, but it usually doesn't. Orthodontic insurance is typically separate from dental insurance, so you should definitely check the details of your dental policy with your insurance provider to find out what's actually covered. If you do get extra insurance to cover orthodontic treatment, you should be aware most policies will come with a lifetime maximum cap of $2,000 that will cover only a portion, or percentage, of the total fee and not 100 percent of your costs. So if your total orthodontic treatment fee is $6,000, your maximum coverage will obviously be $2,000. And the lifetime maximum means the coverage does not renew every year like dental insurance. So you can't get multiple sets of braces and expect coverage for all of them. Some insurance companies require a waiting period too, so if you sign up for new orthodontic insurance, you may have to wait six months before starting orthodontic treatment. Unfortunately, some people aren't aware of this, and they unknowingly start treatment as soon as they get their orthodontic insurance, only to end up forfeiting their coverage. It's also important to understand that most orthodontic insurance will only pay after two years. Say you buy $2,000 in coverage and pay the insurance premium for six months before starting your treatment. If you lose the insurance six months after getting braces, you may only get $500 of what you paid in and you won't get the remaining $1,500. If you end up getting new insurance, they may pick up where the other policy ended, but not all insurance policies will cover work in progress. Some orthodontic insurance also has age limits. So a person over age twenty-one may not be able to get coverage because insurance companies are less likely to cover adult orthodontic treatment.

58. Since I never had braces as a kid, my teeth are gradually getting worse. I'm finally ready to get treatment for myself, but I'm not sure if I

can afford it. Can I pay for my braces with a payment plan, or do I need to pay everything in full?

You won't need to pay the full cost of treatment before you start, and there are many financing options available to you. Fortunately, most orthodontic offices offer payment plans, and you wouldn't have to pay for treatment all at once. In my own office, we typically offer a multiyear installment plan with zero-percent interest, which sometimes extends past your actual treatment time. For instance, your treatment itself might only take a year, but we may extend the payment plan for a period of two years without charging any interest. That means your monthly payments will be lower, and your overall treatment will be more affordable.

Another option is to use an outside company like CareCredit to finance your orthodontic treatment. With CareCredit, you won't have to make any down payment, and you'll have three to four years to pay with a low monthly payment. Although this makes your treatment very affordable, the only downside is that some monthly interest may accrue over the course of your treatment. Many employers offer flexible spending accounts (FSAs) and health savings accounts (HSAs), and these are two good financing alternatives that allow you to benefit from tax deductions by using pretax dollars for your orthodontic treatment. To receive the biggest tax benefit, some people try to use their FSAs to pay for their treatment costs with a lump sum every year. If that's your strategy, be sure to ask your company about enrollment times (the year before treatment) for those plans, so you can get the maximum tax benefits. Even if you don't have an FSA or HSA account, most orthodontists offer a significant discount on the total cost of your treatment if you do choose to pay the full cost of treatment before you start. The bottom line is that most orthodontists offer many different payment options to meet each individual's financial situation to make their treatment more affordable.

59. Without calling a lot of orthodontists, how do I know I'm not being overcharged to get my teeth fixed?

Most orthodontic professionals are honest and won't charge excessively for the treatment they provide. You do, however, need to figure out what their fee includes and what it does not include, because that can make a huge difference in the price of your treatment. Although the fee quoted by one orthodontist may sound a lot higher compared to that charged by others, the higher price may end up being cheaper if it includes everything you'll need.

An all-inclusive fee of $6,700 that covers everything—including braces, breakage of braces, lost appliances, records, extended treatment time, retainers, extra retainers, and clear braces—is probably a better value than a $4,800 fee that doesn't account for any of these extra costs. In fact, you might end up paying far more than $7,000 over the course of three or four years if you add in separate charges for broken braces (which will inevitably happen), retainers (everyone will need a retainer at the end of their treatment), records, extended treatment time (moving teeth takes longer for some patients), clear braces (if you prefer the clear type), or an extra retainer (you may need a replacement retainer in the future). So you may think $6,700 is an overcharge, but in the end, you could save a lot of money with an all-inclusive price, since you'll eventually need to get these extras over the course of your treatment anyway.

That's particularly true if you choose to get Invisalign and have to pay extra every time you lose a tray (which may happen quite often). Since you'll be taking your trays out every time you eat and brush, it's common to forget to put them back in afterward and to leave them behind every now and then. And if you need to get refinement (more Invisalign trays) to keep your teeth aligned, you may incur additional fees unless those fees were included as part of the cost of your treatment package. The same is true of SureSmile or Insignia—a special technology that can give you better and faster treatment results. So if these treatment enhancements are included in your overall fee, you'll be getting a lot more for your money.

60. After I went to see an orthodontist and got a quote for fixing my teeth, I found a second doctor who gave me a much lower quote. Why would there be such a big difference? And why pay more if I can get my teeth straightened more affordably by an orthodontist who will do the work for less?

Seeking and evaluating an orthodontist on the basis of their fees alone isn't a strategy I'd recommend. You may wrongly assume that orthodontics is a commodity, almost like buying a car, but it's definitely not. If you buy a new Honda Accord, for example, you know it's going to be the exact same car wherever you go to buy it, so you'll want to shop around to get the lowest price possible. Unfortunately, not all orthodontists are the same, and the treatment outcomes they provide

> Unfortunately, not all orthodontists are the same, and the treatment outcomes they provide won't be the same either. The skill, experience, responsiveness, and expertise level for each doctor will be different.

won't be the same either. The skill, experience, responsiveness, and expertise level for each doctor will be different. So regarding your price quote, you'd be well advised to do more research to find out why the first orthodontist has quoted a higher price for your treatment. Does he or she offer services that the second person does not? Don't be afraid to contact the first orthodontist to ask tough questions. Time and time again, I've seen patients who went for the cheapest price who had to get braces a second or even third time to get the results they were seeking. Ultimately, evaluating an orthodontist by their fee alone may mean you'll have to pay for treatment twice, and getting the results you deserve may take twice as long. I'm not saying a higher fee necessarily means you're getting a better orthodontist and better outcomes, but you do need to do your research on an orthodontist and find out how long they've been in practice and what aspects of your treatment will be covered by their fee. The first orthodontist you consulted might have been quoting you an all-inclusive fee that covered everything needed for your overall treatment, whereas the second might have been giving you a base cost without the extra charges you'd be likely to incur over the course of your treatment. So don't shop around for an orthodontist based on fees alone. Instead, ask a lot of questions and use your gut feeling after you've gone over all the factors you need to consider.

61. I'm thinking about getting Invisalign because I don't want to wear braces that show. Is Invisalign a lot more expensive than braces?

Invisalign used to be considerably more expensive than traditional metal braces when it first came out more than twenty years ago. Back then, most orthodontists didn't have much experience using this new technology, and because it required more time and effort to get the results metal braces provided, they had to charge more. And although that's still the case for many orthodontists, the cost of Invisalign at my practice is about the same as regular braces (or only slightly higher) for most of my patients. That's because my philosophy as an orthodontist is to guarantee to provide the best treatment possible, and I don't want fees to get in the way of that priority. I understand how important it is for some of my patients to avoid the braces and wires most people associate with the preteen and teen years. And that's what makes Invisalign so perfect for so many. It's not only the most aesthetically pleasing treatment option; it's also the simplest and most convenient one from a hygiene standpoint, since brushing is so much easier. When you stop to think about it, it's actually quite remarkable that just wearing a series of clear removable trays will gradually move your teeth over time. So it's no surprise that Invisalign's popularity is growing. What's frustrating is that many orthodontists still charge more for Invisalign because it raises their overhead. Over the course of treatment, orthodontists have to pay thousands of dollars in lab fees to order Invisalign trays for their patients' changing tooth patterns. Although prices vary between practitioners, these extra lab fees are usually passed on to patients, and that means Invisalign will typically cost you anywhere between $600 and $1,500 more than traditional braces. For many people, the additional cost is well worth it because of the comfort, aesthetics, and lifestyle benefits Invisalign provides.

$62.$ What happens if I move in the middle of my child's orthodontic treatments? I want to start their braces soon, since it's about the right time. But we may be moving to another state in about eight months. Would I get a refund for the fees I've already paid?

If you think you might be moving in less than two years, I'd advise you to hold off and wait until after you've relocated to start your child's orthodontic treatment. Ideally, it's obviously best if you can stay with the same orthodontist from the beginning of your child's treatment until it successfully ends. One of the reasons is that every orthodontist does things slightly differently, and it's most advantageous for your child to work with the same doctor so your child will know what to expect. I work hard to build a relationship of trust with the children I treat, and that trust is an important factor to the good outcomes I see. Consistency is very important to children, and having to adjust to a new doctor in a different orthodontic practice will probably produce some anxiety for them. So unless it's urgent that you start treatment right away, I strongly recommend you wait until you've moved to start braces.

In the event one of my existing patients has to move unexpectedly due to unforeseen circumstances, I prorate their fee based on how much is owed for the work I've already done, and for that work alone. If a patient has already paid in full, I refund all fees for the work I've yet to complete. But you need to know that even after you get that refund, your treatment may end up costing you more, because the new orthodontist may charge additional costs for evaluation and diagnosis before taking you on as a new patient. It's also important to keep in mind that orthodontic fees may vary depending on the location of a practice. The orthodontists in some states and cities charge more than others. So the answer to your question is that most orthodontic offices will work with you to figure out what you've already paid for their completed or planned treatment. But in most cases, you will probably end up paying slightly more than if you were to stay with the same orthodontist.

63. My son started Invisalign treatment about four months ago, but his treatment isn't going well because he's not wearing the trays like he's supposed to. I'm thinking we will have to switch over to braces. I'm scared of having to start all over again. What do you think I should do?

This is a fairly common scenario when working with preteens and teens, so I've mostly stopped charging for a switch in treatment types, and if I charge anything at all, it's just a nominal amount. Although that may sound like a loss for me, I've come to feel it's the right way to handle these kinds of dilemmas. I want my patients and their parents to feel confident that the orthodontic treatment I'm providing is guaranteed to have a successful outcome—and that they're not paying for each appliance, even if a poor outcome is a patient's fault. But in most practices, it doesn't work that way. Unless the possibility of treatment change is spelled out and agreed upon in a contract before starting treatment, you can expect to pay additional costs if you have to change from Invisalign to another treatment option like braces. But even when that's the case, it isn't likely you'd be asked to pay the complete treatment fee all over again but just some portion of the original Invisalign fee to cover the basic Invisalign lab fees or to cover time and material costs for your child's new braces. So you may have to pay some additional charges to switch treatments at most orthodontics offices, but the dirty little secret is that you can always talk to the orthodontist directly, and if you're nice about it, he or she just might be kind enough to override the switch fee.

$64.$ Unfortunately, I lost my retainer at college and stopped wearing it for a few months. I haven't had a chance to go back to my orthodontist yet, and now I'm worried because I've noticed my teeth have shifted. Will I need to get braces all over again?

Losing a retainer is pretty common, and you can simply order a replacement if your teeth haven't shifted too far out of alignment. Once they have, and this best-case-scenario is no longer an option, you can try a special type of retainer called a "spring aligner" to move your teeth back into alignment. This will be the most cost-effective way to realign your teeth. But the downside to this remedial approach is that the appliance itself is quite bulky, and you would have to wear it all the time (literally) for a minimum of six weeks for it to work. If that doesn't sound appealing, your second option is to get braces again. For most people, this may not involve a full set of braces but a limited set for the front six teeth or so. And you should only have to wear them for about three to six months to realign your teeth. That's the good news. The bad news is that you may have to pay 20–40 percent of the total fee you originally paid to have your teeth aligned previously. Your last option would be to get Invisalign. If you had braces before and you would rather get Invisalign for retreatment, this may actually cost you quite a bit more, almost 80 percent of what you would have originally paid for your total braces fee. However, if you initially had Invisalign, and it has been less than five years since you started your original treatment, you could get a substantial discount to do Invisalign all over again, since your case may still be listed as active with the company that made your trays.

65. Is it okay to try to negotiate a reduction in the cost of my orthodontic treatment? How can I qualify to get the maximum discount? Is there a time or season I should start treatment to get the best deal?

If you don't know it already, I want to tell you a really powerful secret: almost anything is negotiable—and that includes the cost of orthodontic treatment. Being a former or active member of the military, a teacher, a health professional, or even a single parent may qualify you for a discount. So will having more than one family member in treatment, something that already qualifies you for a sibling or family discount. And those aren't the only groups and reasons your orthodontist might find it important to give you a discount or a better payment plan. It's also important to know that if you can afford to pay in full and remember to ask for a discount, you may get a substantial one. But please remember you need to be cordial and reasonable when requesting a discount. If you aren't, you may alienate your orthodontist and start your treatment off having a bad relationship with them.

Another valuable secret you need to know is that orthodontic treatment is seasonal. Our busiest time is typically over the summer, and it peaks around August. But the period between September and December tends to be slow since the school year has begun, and most parents and kids aren't interested in starting treatment during this time. That means you may have the most leverage to ask for a discount if you seek orthodontic treatment during a less busy season. It's certainly something to be aware of because many orthodontic practices run seasonal promotions. So if your treatment isn't urgent and it doesn't have to start right away, you should ask the orthodontist if you can wait to benefit from any special promotions they'll be offering in the future. Of course, every orthodontic practice is different, but most do offer some kind of discount, and asking for one isn't something to be embarrassed about!

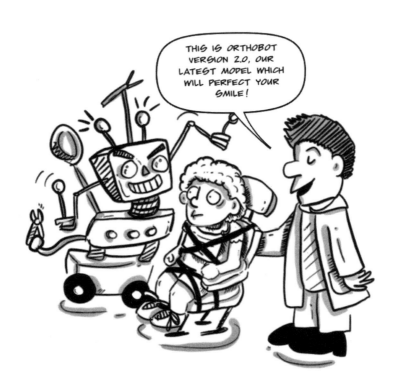

CHAPTER 6

■-■-■-■-■-■-■-■-■

TECHNOLOGY

Thanks to a host of brilliant new innovations in orthodontic technology, you can get your teeth straightened far more quickly and comfortably than ever before. Long gone are the "metal mouth" days of heavy wires and braces that used to be your only option if you wanted to have your teeth fixed. Now you can choose from an array of smaller types of braces and clear aligners, like Invisalign, that use different designs, materials, and colors (or none) that both kids and adults actually like to wear. From your very first evaluation until the day your treatment ends, you'll be enjoying the benefits of orthodontic advances such as digital, 3D x-ray images and digital impression scanners. These scanners are being used in conjunction with computer-aided design (CAD), computer-aided manufacturing (CAM), and robotic wire-bending technology to speed treatment that's far more precise than was ever previously possible. What's even more remarkable is that temporary anchorage devices (TADs) can now enable my patients to bypass jaw surgery they couldn't have avoided in the past. As with the technology transformations in every other field, orthodontic care has gone leading edge with options you might not have heard about yet. Before you start treatment, it's a good idea to know something about these new approaches available to you and to understand a little of how they work.

66. Are today's braces better than the ones people had twenty years ago? If so, how will my sixth-grade son with an overbite benefit from advances in braces technology?

Braces technology has changed a lot in the last two decades, and modern orthodontic treatment offers a vast array of improvements and benefits for both kids and adults alike. Overall, braces are more comfortable, and treatment takes less time, thanks to the variety of new materials now available to orthodontists like me. These days, for example, the individual brackets are placed on the teeth like stickers, making the whole process far more comfortable than it used to be. In the past, the brackets bonded and glued to teeth were much larger, and each tooth had to have a wraparound band, which caused significant discomfort. And the old braces required the use of rubber (elastomer) ties to hold their wires in place. Although it's true those rubber ties are still commonly used today, many orthodontic practices like mine have upgraded to using the new, most advanced braces with gates that open and close. By eliminating the elastomer ties (which can also cause added oral hygiene issues), patients experience less friction between their brackets and wires, and their teeth are freer to shift into alignment more easily. One such bracket used in our office is called the Damon system, and I've found it to be a very effective type of braces treatment—even for patients with orthodontic problems that are typically more difficult to fix.

Metal braces also used to be the only kind available, but they now come in a tooth-colored ceramic type that is less noticeable and more aesthetically pleasing. Of course, the brackets alone can't move and align your teeth. They act as an anchor point for the wires tied to those brackets, making it possible for the wires to exert the pull necessary to gradually straighten your teeth. Like the brackets themselves, these wires have changed. Previously, braces wires were made of stiff steel, but nowadays, these wires are made of light, flexible, incredibly strong nickel titanium, the same material used to make spacecraft at NASA. The lighter and gentler force these wires exert on the teeth allow the bone to adapt better as the teeth are being moved, and they're able to align your teeth with much less discomfort than the older ones made of steel.

67. As a young career woman in my twenties, I don't want braces. What other new orthodontic technologies are available to me if I decide to get my teeth fixed?

If you don't want braces, Invisalign clear aligner therapy is the latest leading-edge treatment for straightening your teeth. This braces-free approach has truly sparked a paradigm shift in the practice of orthodontics, because it's so comfortable, convenient, effective, and aesthetically pleasing. Instead of braces and wires, getting your teeth straightened with Invisalign means you simply wear clear plastic trays that slip over your teeth. Not only that, advances in computer technology have spurred the development of 3D imaging software and x-rays, such as 3D cone beam computed tomography (CBCT) that allows orthodontists to see things we never could in the past. These imaging advances have opened the door to a whole new world of diagnostic vision, where diagnosis and treatment planning can be made with far more accuracy than we once could. Impressionless scanning has also enabled us to create more precise replicas of your teeth without the unpleasant sensation of having molding material in your mouth. That's a big deal for some people, because the feeling of the putty material touching their upper palates can trigger a gag reflex that may cause these patients to throw up, making the whole situation traumatic and messy for them.

SureSmile and Insignia technologies are two other advances that have helped usher in the modern era of customized treatment planning, allowing orthodontists like myself to create the look of each patient's preferred smile. These technologies not only provide better, faster, and more accurate finishes, but they do so while causing less discomfort for my patients and less disruption to their schedules. And thanks to accelerative devices such as Propel VPro5 and AcceleDent, your teeth can be straightened more quickly using micropulsation technology. Both devices emit gentle microvibrations that increase blood flow and cellular activity around your teeth in a way that speeds the rate at which your teeth can move. These portable, convenient, lightweight devices require only a few minutes of daily home use to make treatment time so much faster, that what used to take two or three years can now be done in less than sixteen months. Another benefit of using these devices is pain relief. They reduce discomfort considerably (for both braces and Invisalign), thus making the whole process more comfortable and great for those who are supersensitive to dental procedures. In addition, amazing new Dental Monitoring technology has made it possible for me to check the movements of your teeth remotely. Patients can simply use their cell phones to scan their teeth and upload the scans once a week. The scans are reviewed by the orthodontist, and the progress is digitally compared to the planned movement. Thus, the progress is being carefully monitored even when you are not physically present in the office. In fact, I have several patients traveling from Ohio and Florida and even farther (Los Angeles) and still getting an excellent result using virtual remote monitoring.

68. My college friends keep talking about how happy they are wearing Invisalign instead of braces, and I'm thinking about getting my teeth fixed too. Can you explain how Invisalign works? And what would I have to do to start using it?

Invisalign is an orthodontic treatment approach that people sometimes call "invisible braces." That's a pretty good description since Invisalign straightens your teeth using a series of virtually invisible removable trays you only take out when brushing, eating, or drinking anything (except water). Because each tray is designed to incrementally move your teeth according to a plan designed by your orthodontist, the new trays you receive each week are altered just enough to gradually move your teeth as you wear them every day.

If wearing Invisalign trays sounds easy, you'll be glad to know *starting* Invisalign treatment is simple too. When you come in for your first appointment, I'll scan your teeth using advanced 3D digital software that shows how your teeth will need to be realigned. After your projected treatment plan has been finalized, I'll send the resulting images over to the Invisalign lab, where your weekly trays will be created. Once I've received your trays back from the company, you'll come into the office to try on your first one. You will be asked to wear that first tray for one to two weeks, at least twenty-two hours a day, and then a new tray every week after that. Each week, the different-shaped trays will move your teeth little by little until they've been straightened and moved into their final positions.

Although Invisalign isn't the only company out there that makes the trays—and there are others that offer similar products—I've chosen to use Invisalign exclusively. It is the original company that first developed this novel treatment approach, and I believe it has the best research behind its product and technology. In my office, I also offer accelerative devices such as the Propel VPro5 and AcceleDent, which not only reduce Invisalign treatment time by 30–40 percent but also decrease any soreness related to moving your teeth.

69. I'm a mom of three kids who need braces, but they want Invisalign instead because that's what their friends have. Does Invisalign treatment take longer than traditional braces? Is it okay for all ages?

Like technology in every other medical specialty, Invisalign has been transformed too. And although it's true that Invisalign used to take longer than traditional braces, that's no longer the case. Invisalign now works so well it can align most of my patients' teeth and give them a beautiful, healthy new smile in about the same time, or even a shorter time, than regular braces. What makes that so exciting is that Invisalign is appropriate to use for all ages and is particularly appealing to children. As a matter of fact, you might be surprised to find out that children are often more compliant than adults about wearing their Invisalign trays—because they don't want to have to get metal braces instead. Children's acceptance of Invisalign is extremely important, because it means kids are more likely to get the orthodontic correction they actually need to have healthy teeth. Of course, most adults are enthusiastic about Invisalign too since they don't want to feel embarrassed wearing metal braces around their peers at work.

Treatment time using Invisalign is now comparable to traditional braces thanks to a series of advancements in Invisalign technology. These innovations include the development of AcceleDent that accelerates tooth movement, digital scanning for more accurate impressions, 3D treatment planning, and remote monitoring using Dental Monitoring software, to name just a few. Another reason Invisalign treatment has gotten so much faster is that orthodontists are using better attachments, and the Invisalign company itself has developed more advanced tray materials. Together, these improvements are being used to apply the optimal degree of force needed to create faster, more efficient treatment results using Invisalign. That's terrific news for you if you're like the majority of my patients who are excited to try this great treatment approach to straighten their teeth. The minority who benefit more from traditional braces are those of my patients who have teeth that are severely overcrowded or impacted or that need extraction (before treatment), and regular braces are still better suited to fix their teeth in terms of speed and result.

70. When I go online, I keep seeing offers for mail-order aligner treatment. Is this an option that's as safe and effective as getting Invisalign through an orthodontist?

Mail-order orthodontic treatment as a do-it-yourself (DIY) service is a relatively new phenomenon. Although it's probably obvious to most people, the problem with this approach is that orthodontics is a rather complex medical specialty that requires many years of postgraduate education to master. Treatment skills have to be proven before an orthodontist's credentials are awarded by established medical institutions. I don't know about you, but if I were a surgeon, I wouldn't want to do surgery on my own body, just by watching YouTube videos that show how it's done. You need to have someone knowledgeable monitor the changes in your teeth and jaw, and you need to be able to consult with an expert who will be responsible for the success of your treatment. In other words, you are taking a risk trying to undertake aligner treatment by yourself.

Teeth don't always move as planned, and if something goes wrong, you will be on your own. I'm not saying there's absolutely no market for this. These DIY treatments may work for cases requiring minor adjustments, and you may save a few bucks. And things may work out for you if you try this kind of self-treatment, but when they don't, you'll have to pay a big price for your mistake. It's my professional opinion that the trial-and-error approach isn't advisable when it comes to orthodontic treatment, since the potential risk usually outweighs the benefit. A noted problem with Generation Z kids between ages twenty and twenty-four is that they have little aversion to risk. Convenience, instant gratification, and lower costs can be sufficient motivation for them to risk a dangerous, lifelong, and irreversible outcome. Likewise, you're obviously risking the proper alignment of your jaw and teeth if you decide to self-administer aligner treatment—

> The trial-and-error approach isn't advisable when it comes to orthodontic treatment, since the potential risk usually outweighs the benefit.

so I certainly wouldn't advise you to try this DIY approach.

71. Since I'm getting married in eight months, I want to start and finish my braces within that time period. Is there a way to accelerate my treatment? If so, are there any risks to doing it faster?

There are a variety of ways to accelerate your orthodontic work and reduce your treatment time before big life events. Whether it can be done in as little as eight months depends on the position of your individual teeth and your jaw alignment, because complex problems simply require more time. So your first step is to be evaluated by an orthodontist as soon as possible. If I was the orthodontist you came to see, I'd want to tell you about all the accelerative strategies I can use to speed your braces treatment.

Your first option is to use a special type of self-ligating braces that have small built-in latches that open and close as needed. Self-ligating braces work faster than the traditional ones (that stay open all the time) because they don't create as much of the friction that slows down the movement of your teeth as they're being aligned. The friction generated by traditional braces stems from having to secure wires to the always-open braces with a great number of rubber ties. With self-ligating braces, however, the built-in latch eliminates the need for rubber ties altogether, and the wires can just slide along the braces.

The second way I can accelerate your treatment is by using a digital imaging system to create custom-made brackets and wires that will move your teeth more quickly than standard braces. The two most popular types are Insignia, where the brackets are custom cut and designed for each patient, and SureSmile, where the wire is custom created with robotic technology. By using these computer and robotic innovations, your teeth can be safely and successfully moved with increased precision and speed.

A third alternative to a faster treatment outcome is to use a special handheld device such as VPro5 or AcceleDent that uses mechanical pulsations to stimulate your teeth to move into alignment more quickly. Whichever one you choose, this approach requires you to simply hold either of these orthodontic devices between your teeth anywhere from five to twenty minutes a day. The micropulsations they emit create vibrational forces in your teeth and bone, which activate specialized cells that encourage your teeth to move more quickly than normal braces can by themselves. If that sounds like science fiction, it may reassure you to know this technology was first used by orthopedic surgeons to speed up the healing process of bone fractures by applying these kinds of pulsating vibrations.

As another alternative, I offer a fourth treatment choice called micro-osteoperforation (MOP) to accelerate tooth movement and hasten alignment. This approach stimulates faster bone development by using a Propel device to create extremely tiny punctures in the bone around the teeth. Although that may sound painful, it's really not, so the MOP procedure is typically done using topical anesthesia, and no needles or shots are even needed.

72. Can accelerated orthodontic treatment harm my children's teeth in any way? Won't moving teeth too fast cause serious problems?

Accelerated treatment doesn't necessarily mean I'm moving your teeth faster by increasing the pressure on your teeth. I know that probably sounds confusing, so let me explain. Self-ligating brackets, for example, help your teeth move more efficiently because they create less friction than traditional brackets. To get an idea of what I mean, imagine you're moving a big refrigerator by pushing it along the floor. This generates a lot of friction that slows its movement, requiring you to exert more force to keep it going. But imagine what would happen if you spread oil on the floor, or even better, put wheels on the bottom of that refrigerator. Doing so will decrease friction and allow you to push the refrigerator much more quickly even though you're using less force. So please remember that opting to use an accelerated orthodontic treatment doesn't mean I'll be moving your teeth "harder" and with more force—which can definitely be a bad thing for your teeth. Applying too much force with braces will certainly lead to problems, which is why accelerated approaches rely on using a lighter force to get teeth moving. Accelerative techniques actually allow me to move your teeth faster, but more gently, while using less force to achieve optimal treatment results.

A second reason these techniques deliver better, quicker results is because new innovative computer technologies such as SureSmile enable me to customize treatments with far more directional precision than I could in the past. Remember my refrigerator analogy? Even less friction won't help if you're moving that refrigerator in the wrong direction and you haven't lined it up correctly to get it through a doorway. Using SureSmile's computerized system allows me to custom create wires that can move your unique teeth in the direction they need to go with greater precision. So SureSmile moves the teeth faster and shortens treatment time by applying pressure more accurately and "aiming" the teeth more precisely. Think about it. When you get somewhere faster using your GPS device, it isn't because you drove more rapidly but because you used the best route—the one that was most direct and precise—to get to your destination.

73. My coworker told me about SureSmile technology, but she didn't tell me what it is or how it works. Can you explain how this technology is different from normal braces and how it can benefit me when I get braces?

Orthodontic treatment with SureSmile technology uses a fundamentally different approach from traditional braces, and that's obvious from the outset. Your treatment would begin by creating a digital 3D computer model of your teeth that's used to interface with complex computer software. This software is able to analyze the digital 3D model of your teeth and measure the position and angle of each tooth with incredible precision. When you start traditional braces, however, your orthodontist won't be able to measure your teeth in this precise way but will just be eyeballing it with visual observation. Because they can't really tell if your tooth is angled one way at five degrees or eight degrees, that lack of data means pressure can't be applied in just the right place. But using SureSmile allows an orthodontist to do just that: it provides extremely accurate measurements that form the basis of a virtual treatment plan created from computer algorithms. These software-sourced treatment plans determine how, and where, to apply pressure most precisely to move each of your teeth most effectively and efficiently. Each of these detailed movements is then transferred to robotic technology in which a robotic arm is used to precisely bend the braces wires with far more accuracy than any human could—including the most skilled orthodontist in the world. This accuracy is a really big deal, because in braces treatment, the wire is more important than the braces themselves. The wires are the component of braces that actually move the teeth, while each bracket merely acts as a kind of handle, or attachment point, for those wires.

When wires created by SureSmile are inserted into a bracket, they will move the teeth with far more precision than was ever possible before, because they're custom created for each individual. The benefit to you is fewer appointments, shorter treatment time, less overall discomfort, and higher-quality results than traditional braces can offer. Perhaps best of all, SureSmile technology allows an orthodontist to custom create smiles that are uniquely suited to each individual from the very outset of treatment.

74. Although I understand how SureSmile works, I don't want to pay more for my daughter's braces. Why should I pay extra when regular braces will give her the same results?

It's true that opting to use SureSmile braces may cost you $1,500 to $2,000 more than traditional braces in many orthodontic offices. But even when that's the case, I think SureSmile is worth the extra expense for several key reasons. Perhaps the most important one is that I believe you should have to get braces only once. I've seen some patients who had braces previously, but the way their teeth looked afterward wasn't what they expected, and they ended up coming to see me and having to pay to get braces a second time. Personally, I'd rather have treatment that gave me a smile I loved the first time around instead of hoping to achieve better results after a second attempt. Another reason I'm convinced SureSmile is worth the money is that the little subtleties of correct alignment and finish may not seem important to you now, but they can have long-term and far-reaching effects down the road. Wearing braces for a much shorter time (about 30 percent less) means less chance of decay and healthier gums during treatment. And getting better angulation of your teeth and bite is something that will affect and benefit you for the rest of your life. That's because the straighter your teeth, the less likely you are to suffer from the gum disease that causes receding gums or even bone loss due to gingivitis or periodontal disease later in life. In other words, subtle discrepancies in tooth alignment may not have an immediate effect on you now, but in the long term, they most certainly could.

In my own orthodontic office, the SureSmile fee is comparable to traditional braces, or in some cases, just slightly higher by $400–$600 over the regular braces fee. I price it this way because the technology is so effective, I want it to be available to as many people as possible. I believe focusing on providing a better outcome for my patients is an approach that does far more to market my reputation as an orthodontist than worrying about losing a bit in overhead does. In fact, other than the high price some offices charge for SureSmile, I don't see any other downside to using it. But it's important for you to realize that SureSmile is just a tool, and its success will depend on how much experience an orthodontist has using it. Personally, I've treated more than three thousand patients using SureSmile over the last ten years or so. So if you want to use SureSmile, you might want to find an orthodontist who has been using it for a while on a lot of their patients. You'll also want to verify you won't be charged a big difference between SureSmile and traditional braces.

75. Is it worth it to try to find an orthodontist who is using the new 3D x-ray machines? Can 3D imaging really help my family's orthodontic treatments have a better outcome than 2D imaging?

Many of my patients mistakenly think the panoramic x-ray machine in my orthodontic office that takes 2D panoramic and cephalometric x-rays is taking 3D images because of the way the panoramic x-ray tube moves around their heads. But that's not the case. I have to explain that, until recently, most orthodontists have had to rely on 2D x-rays to diagnose their patients' teeth and jaw issues. But that's all changed now. Thanks to recent advancements in imaging technology, I can offer 3D cone beam computed tomography (CBCT) right in my office via our i-CAT FLX x-ray machine. While a patient is seated, the i-CAT FLX CBCT scanner rotates once around them, using a cone-shaped x-ray beam to collect the data needed to create 3D images. This incredible device produces highly accurate 3D images that allow me to view a patient's mouth, teeth, jaw, and sinuses in unprecedented detail—yet it emits radiation comparable to that of a traditional panoramic x-ray machine.

The 3D CBCT x-rays have opened up a whole new world for orthodontists. Seeing so much that wasn't previously visible has equipped us to devise more effective treatment plans and produce better results than ever before. These 3D images allow me to measure the airways of

> The 3D CBCT x-rays have opened up a whole new world for orthodontists. Seeing so much that wasn't previously visible has equipped us to devise more effective treatment plans and produce better results than ever before.

my patients, for example, to check for decreased airway volume or other serious undiagnosed airway problems—issues that could ultimately prove life threatening in both children and adults if they're not treated. When that's the case, the clear view provided by 3D imaging enables me to devise an effective treatment plan for airway problems using intraoral devices or by referring patients to the right specialist. What's more, 3D images allow me to detect and assess skeletal problems more accurately. If a patient's upper or lower jaw is positioned too far to one side, for example, 3D images allow me to measure the deviation more precisely so I can create the best possible treatment plan and outcome.

I'm also able to diagnose patients' temporomandibular joint (TMJ) dysfunctions without any guesswork, because the newer 3D images enable me to see their TMJ so clearly. Thanks to these images, I can check the exact position of patients' individual teeth, and if one of them is impacted, it's far easier to correctly determine whether to remove it or to lower it with treatment. 3D imaging also allows me to detect abnormalities and problems I wouldn't be able to see by taking regular 2D x-rays, like detecting an extra tooth hidden between two other teeth below the gumline. And being able to plan the movement of the roots for each tooth in 3D view means I get more precise finishes when such planning is used in conjunction with SureSmile. Perhaps most startling of all, I've unexpectedly detected malignancies in adult patients with 3D imaging and been able to refer them to an oral surgeon for treatment before the cancer spread further. And there have been countless times I've found cysts in children, such as traumatic bone cysts on their lower jaws, that I might have missed altogether using traditional 2D x-rays.

76. Radiation exposure from 3D x-rays is a big concern for me, so I don't want to have a CT taken for braces treatment. Is my concern justified or not?

Just about everyone's had dental x-rays, and most of the people who have gotten them realize they've been exposed to some radiation in the process. So it only makes sense to find out what's considered a safe exposure level, especially for newer imaging technologies. That's why it's important for you to understand that the 3D cone beam computed tomography (CBCT) I use to plan your orthodontic treatment is not the same as medical computed tomography (CT). Medical CT exams expose you to vastly more radiation than CBCT exams because CT creates a wide fan of x-ray beams to create true 3D images. CBCT, on the other hand, uses a much narrower and more focused cone-shaped beam instead. It does not actually take real 3D images like medical CT scans do, but it captures 2D images from varying angles and then reconstructs them into a 3D image.

The ionizing radiation emitted by medical and dental x-rays are measured in units called microsieverts to express how much radiation your body is actually absorbing. Our CBCT machine (i-CAT FLX) will only expose you to anywhere between 5.3 and 8.5 microsieverts during a typical scanning—unless I need to do more detailed scanning, which might increase your exposure to 12–25 micro-sieverts. But these scans are usually done only at the very beginning and the very end of your orthodontic treatment. Since the newest i-CAT FLX CBCT scanning actually emits less radiation than tradi-tional 2D panoramic x-rays for a typical scanning, you can be assured scanning exposes you to a very minimal amount.

Having explained that, I realize this information really doesn't tell you much. So just to give you some perspective on the question of radiation exposure in the US, you'll be interested to know your exposure to typical background radiation is around 8 microsieverts per day. And flying from New York City to San Francisco will subject you to about 40–60 additional microsieverts. In comparison, a typical scanning performed with an i-CAT FLX CBCT machine in my office emits only 5.3–8.5 microsieverts, which means the dose you would receive is negligible. Even so, I use a treatment approach that minimizes the need to take x-rays as much as possible. But when I do take x-rays, my staff and I use proper protective measures, including a lead apron that covers your whole upper body up to the neck. We also conduct yearly calibration and testing of our machines, and the x-ray badges worn by our staff are measured monthly.

77. I don't like having molding material in my mouth because it makes me gag, so I'm relieved to hear some orthodontists are using a new kind of impressionless scanning. Does this kind of scanner emit radiation?

An impressionless scanner (iTero Element intraoral scanner) isn't an x-ray machine, and it emits zero radiation, so you don't have to worry about any radiation risks when you have your impressions made with the device. This intraoral (inside-the-mouth) digital scanner takes 3D images of your teeth and records the data using computer software. An important orthodontic tool, these images are essential for diagnostic purposes or to fabricate different devices (retainers, expanders, Invisalign) that will fit your unique teeth and bite configuration better than ever before. Most people would agree impressionless scanning is a big improvement over the way impressions (dental molds) have traditionally been made—a process requiring patients to bite into putty material during a procedure that causes some people to gag and throw up. It also makes many of my patients feel they can't breathe, and some have actually suffered panic attacks because of that fear.

The new impressionless process is so much more comfortable for my patients. When a digital intraoral scanner is used to make your molds, a small wand is simply waved across your teeth while you're seated in a chair. As the wand passes over your teeth (not touching your teeth) it captures thousands of images each second. That's all there is to it! During scanning, you can breathe and swallow as you normally would. And the whole process is so fast, it takes less than three minutes. The images are combined to create a 3D digital model of your teeth that's far more accurate than any model made with putty impression material. Plus, the 3D images of your teeth are created instantly, so your orthodontist can immediately show you the results of your planned treatment. You can even view computer-generated simulations of your before and after outcomes right then and there! Not only that, your impressionless digital scans are sent instantly via the internet, which means a rapid turnaround time for Invisalign trays. That's so much better than having to send out the traditional putty impressions by mail, which unavoidably delays the start of treatment.

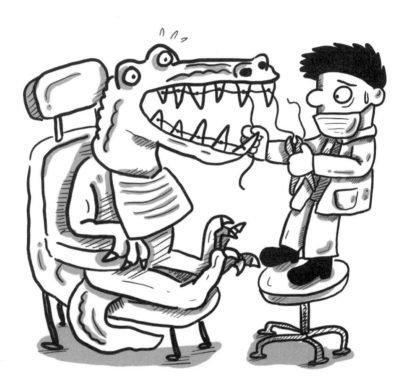

CHAPTER 7

NONTRADITIONAL TREATMENT

N ontraditional orthodontics can truly change the lives of the adults and children I see who have restricted airways and temporomandibular joint issues caused by a narrow jaw or bad bite. Yet most of these patients are surprised to find out the position of their teeth and bite, or the size of their jaw, is somehow linked to their health problems—disorders such as mouth breathing, sleep apnea, snoring, tooth grinding, chronic headaches, and even behavioral or learning difficulties. Believe it or not, all of those different problems are often connected to a patient's restricted airway hampering their ability to breathe normally, or to a bad bite causing abnormal tension and function of their jaw joint. Like my other patients with these issues, you'll be relieved to know I can use nontraditional orthodontic approaches to greatly improve, or even resolve, these serious health concerns. One of the nontraditional treatments I've found effective for widening airways, for example, is the rapid palatal expander (RPE) that can expand a narrow jaw to facilitate better breathing. And to keep airways open during sleep, I may have patients wear intraoral devices that look like a special kind of mouth guard. I can also use temporary anchorage devices (TADs), or miniscrews, to correct a variety of jaw problems that used to require jaw surgery. What's more, I'm able to conduct TruDenta evaluations and therapy to better assess patients' bites in a way that often enables me to resolve the headache and jaw pain caused by constricted facial muscles. For those with bruxism, I can prescribe special night guards to prevent tooth grinding during sleep. Perhaps most amazing of all, I can use remote Dental Monitoring to check to see if your treatment is working as planned from wherever you happen to be when you use the app on your smartphone. Since nontraditional orthodontic treatments can offer so much relief from the lifelong health problems linked to poor breathing or a bad bite, it's wise to find out how they can help you too.

78. Will orthodontic treatment help with mouth breathing? I've noticed my child has a hard time breathing through his nose, and he's constantly walking around with his mouth open. Won't that predispose him to having more cavities since it dries out his mouth?

Orthodontics can help stop your child's mouth breathing if the problem is happening because the roof (palate) of their mouth is too narrow—a characteristic that often restricts a child's upper airways too. Working with an orthodontist to correct that issue is very important. Doing so not only helps prevent dental decay and gum inflammation but also protects your child from a variety of serious health problems. When a child can't breathe normally through their nose, for example, they'll often grind, gnash, or clench their teeth (bruxism), which not only wears down their tooth surfaces but causes sleep problems—something that can negatively affect every aspect of their lives. What's more, mouth breathing can produce an abnormal bite or atypical jaw development in a child who is constantly holding their mouth open. And mouth breathing may even be the reason your child is getting sick more easily. Instead of inhaling warmed, purified air through their nose, they're breathing cold, unfiltered air that's still full of the allergens and infection-causing microorganisms the nose is meant to filter out.

Although your child's mouth breathing may stem from something other than having a narrow palate—including nasal obstructions, sinus issues, or adenoid and tonsil problems—it's vital you have an orthodontist check to find out. In fact, this is something I assess during a child's first evaluation at my own orthodontic practice. If I see a child has a narrow palate and isn't breathing through their nose normally, I can usually correct that by seating an expander device in the roof of their mouth. This simple, lightweight frame will widen their palate and their upper jaw with gentle pressure. By creating more space in the child's upper airway, this treatment can correct a child's mouth-breathing issues if it's done early enough, before the two sections of their upper palate fuse around age twelve. After that, widening a narrow jaw will require jaw surgery, so it's very important to have your child evaluated by an orthodontist as soon as you begin seeing them start mouth breathing regularly. In some cases, widening their upper palate won't be enough, and their adenoids or tonsils will need to be removed to free up their lower airway. In such cases, I refer my patients to an ear, nose, and throat doctor.

79. Can orthodontic treatment help my sleep apnea get better or go away completely? My doctor referred me to an orthodontist after telling me I have the condition, but how is sleep apnea related to my teeth?

When a person has sleep apnea, they temporarily stop breathing for ten to thirty seconds at a time while sleeping. That may not seem like much, but since it can happen multiple times a night, the lost sleep will obviously hamper your school or work productivity. And the negative health effects can range from having a headache or being tired and grouchy to pulmonary hypertension—a serious condition characterized by high blood pressure in the arteries leading to the lungs. The most common type of sleep apnea is called obstructive sleep apnea (OSA). Other types include central sleep apnea and complex sleep apnea syndrome. But since you can't determine which kind you have on your own, you'll have to check back with your physician to find out.

If you have the OSA type, it means something is blocking your airway and making it more difficult for you to breathe. OSA has been linked to high blood pressure and other health problems, and it can be life threatening in its most severe form. The obstruction blocking your airway can be caused either by soft tissue in your throat or by your tongue or jaw being positioned too far back. If you're like most people, your physician probably diagnosed it by having you get a sleep test done, either at a sleep study facility or by taking a home sleep test.

Once you've been diagnosed with OSA, there are several solutions. In some cases, surgery may be needed, but most commonly, a continuous positive airway pressure (CPAP) machine or intraoral (inside-the-mouth) device is used. By blowing air into your mouth, a CPAP machine forcibly opens up your airway. This approach works great, but the compliance rate using the machine is very low because many people find it uncomfortable to sleep hooked up to the machine while wearing a full or partial mask attached to an air hose. If you can't tolerate a CPAP machine, you should ask your orthodontist to fit you with an intraoral (inside the mouth) device that looks like a mouth guard. Wearing one of these at night will help hold your airway open by keeping the position of your lower jaw moved forward while you're sleeping, so you can breathe more freely.

Fortunately, compliance using intraoral devices is quite high, and most of my patients who use them enjoy improved sleep patterns. I'm glad that's the case because I know getting better sleep means their overall immunity will be higher, and they'll be better able to fight off disease. By getting more complete rest, my patients find they feel better emotionally, have more energy, and enjoy a better ability to concentrate during the day. They tell me they can perform better at work and at school and suffer fewer of the headaches and muscle aches associated with poor sleep.

Since so many car accidents occur as a result of falling asleep at the wheel while driving, CPAP or intraoral devices should be considered a lifesaving treatment. When left untreated, the more severe forms of sleep apnea can lead to myriad health issues, and in the worst cases, cause strokes

> When left untreated, the more severe forms of sleep apnea can lead to myriad health issues, and in the worst cases, cause strokes and heart attacks to occur during sleep. So you should take a diagnosis of sleep apnea very seriously, since the condition can lead to a life-or-death situation.

and heart attacks to occur during sleep. So you should take a diagnosis of sleep apnea very seriously, since the condition can lead to a life-or-death situation. With that in mind, there are relational benefits too. Most people with sleep apnea will snore, and if your snoring is loud, it can obviously affect the sleep of your spouse—even forcing them to sleep in a separate room—which can lead to marital strain. As you might imagine, treating an OSA with an intraoral device would be a much better solution relationally, as it promotes better health for everyone involved.

$80.$ Since my daughter snores, I'm worried that's a sign she may have an airway obstruction. Can braces help with this?

Snoring doesn't necessarily mean your child has obstructive sleep apnea (OSA), but it can certainly be an indication that they do. So you should definitely check with their physician to determine whether your child's snoring is related to OSA, since lack of sleep can actually affect your child's growth and development. Although traditional braces treatment won't alleviate OSA, I can (and often do) use a rapid palatal expander (RPE) device for three to six months to help widen a child's narrow upper airway, a strategy that can alleviate their breathing problems during sleep. The reason this often works is that the two distinct growth plates in the roof (palate) of a child's mouth can be widened if their upper jaw is too narrow—or their airway is restricted and causing OSA. I can solve the problem by fitting a child with a simple lightweight RPE that uses gentle pressure to gradually spread apart the two halves of their palate. This widens their upper jaw and their airway at the same time, and that extra space creates more airway for them to breathe through.

Using the upper molars as anchors, the expander is seated in such a way that it produces a gentle tension that steadily separates the suture in the middle of the palate where the child's two growth plates meet. Since a child's suture won't fuse together until they're eleven or twelve, this process shouldn't hurt at all. Thanks to the effectiveness of this simple device, I've personally seen expanders help many kids with airway issues. It's remarkable that so many lifelong benefits can be gained with this simple nonsurgical approach. After getting expander therapy to widen their upper jaws and airways (and sometimes in combination with the removal of their tonsils or adenoids), a lot of the kids I see with OSA symptoms have their symptoms completely disappear. That means they no longer snore, wake up at night, or experience night terrors—which means they can sleep better, so they're no longer tired during the day. And when I talk to the moms of those kids, many tell me their children are breathing and sleeping so much better, they start behaving better at school and at home—two things that are directly linked in a way many health practitioners miss.

I'm gratified that diagnosing OSA has gotten much easier too, thanks to recent technological breakthroughs in 3D imaging with cone beam computed tomography (CBCT) x-ray machines. CBCT images allow me to measure a child's airway before and after expander treatment, and such images conclusively show how significantly expanders widen airways. Sometimes I see kids whose initial imaging shows their airway problem might be related to enlarged adenoids or tonsils, in which case I typically refer them to an ear, nose, and throat (ENT) physician. After evaluating a child with this issue, an ENT might recommend their adenoids or tonsils be removed—which should greatly improve the function of their airway.

81. I was told that sleep apneas can sometimes lead to symptoms of ADHD in children. I've also heard that orthodontic treatment can help improve ADHD behaviors. Is this true?

When a child has obstructive sleep apnea (OSA), it can prevent them from getting enough rest because their impaired breathing prevents them from entering a full deep sleep and cycling through the five ninety-minute sleep stages that characterize a normal night's sleep. If you see your child stop breathing for a few seconds, or if they habitually snore when they're sleeping, it could mean they have OSA. And that's a serious problem because having OSA means your child won't be getting the rest their body desperately needs. You probably already know that kids need more sleep than adults, but you may not know why. The reason is that children are developing very rapidly, but their bodies secrete the growth hormone they require for their rapid development only while they're asleep. So when OSA prevents a child from getting the full rest they need, they tend to feel agitated. To stay awake during the day, they may have to stay constantly active to fight their need for sleep. Every parent with a normal overly tired toddler is familiar with this kind of pattern. Instead of winding down when they're tired, they just get more wound up and agitated.

The same thing happens with older kids too. Sleep deficiencies can lead to behaviors that look very similar to attention deficit hyperactivity disorder (ADHD) because they can impair a child's ability to learn. Sometimes kids are even misdiagnosed as having ADHD when their symptoms are actually due to sleep deficiency. It's easy to see why. Children with abnormal, disrupted sleep tend to become restless and unable to concentrate during the day, because they're not getting enough of the oxygen and growth hormones they need to grow and function properly. It's troubling that a misdiagnosis of

ADHD means a child will probably be medicated throughout their school and college years for a condition they don't actually have. Since all medications have the potential for side effects, coupling these with years of poor sleep during your child's developmental years means your child would be exposed to serious life-affecting physical, mental, and emotional dangers that could have been avoided.

But thankfully, you can do something about it. In my own orthodontic practice, for example, I use a palate expander device that gently and painlessly widens a child's upper jaw over the course of three to six months. This approach, when combined with adenoids or tonsils removal, can resolve your child's OSA because widening their palate also opens up their airways so they can breathe better. By treating OSA, a lot of kids I see with an ADHD diagnosis are able to focus so much better, and their ADHD symptoms "magically" disappear.

82. My orthodontist said I need jaw surgery. But when I went for a second opinion, I was told that I can be treated with miniscrews instead of surgery. What is miniscrew treatment, and how does it work?

A miniscrew is actually a temporary anchorage device (TAD), and it's something an orthodontist can use to effectively treat some of their most complex cases. TADs are basically small screws or plates I place on strategic places between the teeth or upper palate. Because they act like a solid anchor, I can use them to selectively move teeth, close spaces where implants would have been needed before, or align the symmetry of the upper jaw where one side is lower than the other side. In fact, this approach works so well, I no longer have to refer my patients with open bites to oral surgeons for jaw surgery. Instead,

I can correct the problem using miniscrews and braces to "intrude" (or partially move) their back molars into the bone beneath them. TADs are an amazing technological development in patient care, and in my own practice, I now successfully use them to correct the complicated kinds of orthodontic problems I never would have imagined I could fix with braces alone. It's actually become routine for me to use a combination of braces and TADs to treat patients that used to require jaw surgery or an implant. In my practice, I place the TADs myself after applying a topical (gel) anesthesia to the gum tissue without using any needles.

83. Do you think my severe headaches could be linked to my bad bite? I've tried everything, but nothing seems to be working, and sometimes I can barely stand the pain at my job. Could orthodontic treatment help?

I'm sure you already know that headaches can be triggered by many different factors. But what you may not realize is that research suggests chronic migraines and tension headaches may be caused by the same thing triggering vertigo and tinnitus—temporomandibular joint dysfunction (TMD) of the temporomandibular joint—and that all of these conditions may be interconnected.[1] The fact that TMD triggers pain in the face, jaw, and neck, for example, points to the fact that all of these conditions have something in common: they lead to changes in specific nerves and set off chemical reactions that result in chronic pain. It's understandable why alleviating chronic pain is

---

1   See, for instance, Amira Mokhtar Abouelheda et al., "Association between Headache and Temporomandibular Disorder," *Journal of the Korean Association of Oral and Maxillofacial Surgeons* December 2017, 43(6): 363–367; Pamela Maria Kusdra et al., "Relationship between Otological Symptoms and TMD," *Int Tinnitus J*, June 2018, 22(1): 30-34.

the focus of treating these disorders, but in doing so, the underlying *causes* of that pain have been largely ignored. Although various pills can provide some short-term pain relief to make these conditions more bearable day to day, relying on this approach as a long-term strategy will actually perpetuate the pain and headaches you want to eliminate. That's why identifying the source of your condition is so crucial, and working with an orthodontist is a good place to start.

The reason an orthodontist might be able to help resolve your chronic headaches is because they could be related to a bad bite or a dysfunction in the way your jaws fit together, as with TMD. If your bite is off, your jaw joint won't intersect properly, which can cause persistent muscle tension that eventually builds into the pain of chronic headaches. Conventional orthodontic treatment can address this problem by aligning your teeth and correcting your bad bite (if you have one). Once that's done, you may be surprised to find that fixing these two issues has resolved your headaches too. The reason for this outcome can be explained by the fact that muscles damaged with scar tissue can also create the trigger points that have been implicated as a cause of chronic headaches. We now know, for example, that the nerves in the part of the brain linked to headache pain are the same as those that create dental pain. In other words, nerves that serve the muscles of the mouth and jaw are located in the nerve center that causes headaches too. That's why resolving trigger points and muscle spasms around the mouth and jaw is ground zero for treating your chronic headaches. And that's where a therapy called TruDenta can help.

I offer TruDenta therapy in my orthodontic practice because I've found it to be a very effective way to eliminate the chronic headaches of patients who are searching for long-term pain relief. If that's you, I'd like to explain what you can expect if you come in for treatment.

I start by conducting detailed diagnostic tests that precisely measure any imbalances in the way your teeth and bite come together. This complete battery of tests individualizes your treatment and is one of the reasons TruDenta has proven to be such an effective rehabilitative approach. During the T-Scan test, for example, I measure your bite force and create a unique 3D map of your mouth that's so precise, it shows where each individual tooth is exerting force. I'll also evaluate your jaw's range of motion and alignment. Once I've compiled the results of these assessments, I'm able to diagnose the headache-related muscular issues I'll need to address with TruDenta.

The therapy itself involves four treatment modalities: cold laser therapy, manual muscle therapy, microcurrent therapy, and ultrasound therapy. Cold laser therapy is applied first to decrease your pain and inflammation, accelerate the healing of jaw muscle tissue, and reconnect the neurological pathways of nerves connecting to the brain stem. Manual muscle therapy is used next to decrease the intensity of trigger points and eliminate them by breaking up muscle knots and increasing blood flow. Afterward, microcurrent therapy is employed to relax jaw muscle spasms that refer pain, to decrease lactic acid buildup, and to encourage healthy nerve stimulation. Last of all, ultrasound therapy is used to bring circulation back into sore, strained jaw muscles and break up scar tissue with vibration that penetrates deeply into your muscles. All these modalities are designed to specifically target and resolve the muscle issues causing your headaches. And they work!

84. My daughter's jaws make a popping sound when she opens her mouth, and she says there's a place just below her ear that's started

hurting. Could this be a problem orthodontics could relieve, and if not, is it likely to get worse as she gets older?

What you're describing sounds like temporomandibular joint (TMJ) dysfunction, or TMD, although I'd need to evaluate your daughter to tell for sure. As an orthodontist, I can tell you the TMD issue is three to four times more common in females than males, and the reason for that difference is thought to be related to female hormone levels. That's probably why the symptoms of this jaw disorder typically crop up first during the teen years, between ages twelve and fifteen. Heredity seems to play a strong role in TMD as well, and if a mom has it, there's a fair chance her daughter may have it too. Although there's a strong genetic component to TMD, having a bad bite just exacerbates the situation and creates muscle imbalances that affect the position of the jaw joint.

If a person's jaw joint makes only a slight clicking or popping sound when it moves, it shouldn't be a big cause for concern—just as it is normal for a person's knees to make a popping noise when they bend over and for people to "crack" their knuckles. But when the clicking or popping is present in a jaw that locks up, can't open and close normally, or can't move without pain—and any of those symptoms is coupled with headaches—these are signs of full-blown TMD. To diagnose this conclusively, I use a special CBCT x-ray machine that creates detailed 3D images of the joint so I can get a clear idea of the TMJ's position to determine whether there is actual physical deterioration of the joint.

Because I was trained in the Roth/Williams course for ongoing orthodontic issues, I use special dental equipment called an articulator to accurately assess the true position of a person's bite. Once that's been determined and a proper diagnosis has been made, I will start orthodontic treatment to correct a patient's bite. In conjunction with fixing their jaw alignment, I will also want to restore the health of the patient's muscle tissue by using TruDenta therapy. As a last step, I would need to check a patient for airway issues and sleep apnea, since sleep apnea can cause the muscle tension that sometimes leads to TMD issues.

85. Our thirteen-year-old son has been grinding his teeth in his sleep since childhood, and we'd like to know if braces can fix the problem, since we know it can damage his teeth long term. If not, do you recommend we have a custom night guard made for him, or can he use an over-the-counter night guard?

Braces can help stop tooth grinding (also known as bruxism) when a misaligned jaw or teeth are causing the problem. The fact that your son is grinding his teeth when he's sleeping is a good indicator an abnormal bite or crooked teeth are indeed to blame. But since those issues are just two of the many factors that can trigger bruxism, you should definitely have him checked by an orthodontist to find out if that's actually the case. Most practices don't charge a fee for initial consultations like this, and an orthodontist will have the required expertise to determine if bite issues are causing the tooth grinding you're concerned about. If it's any consolation, bruxism affects 14–17 percent of all children, and about a third of those kids will still be grinding their teeth as adults. Since your son is obviously one of them, it

> Bruxism affects 14–17 percent of all children, and about a third of those kids will still be grinding their teeth as adults.

would be wise to check into the underlying cause of his bruxism, so you can find a solution that will protect his teeth from the damage it is doing to his tooth enamel. It isn't meant to withstand the constant, prolonged pressure of his clenched teeth grinding against each other for hours at a time. This tooth grinding is nothing like the rhythmic, periodic pressure teeth experience during eating (which doesn't usually hurt them at all). Of course, that's assuming your son isn't habitually eating ice or chomping down on jawbreakers or other rock-hard food items!

The reason a bad bite leads to tooth grinding is because it often causes jaw muscle strain as the body tries to remedy the misalignment by self-adjusting the position of the jaw. That doesn't really work and causes problems over time. Like two big puzzle pieces, a person's upper and lower jaw (and teeth) have to meet and fit together perfectly for them to function properly. When they don't, the jaw joint can become displaced as the body tries to compensate by getting the teeth to align better. Many years of this unconscious self-adjustment can create a discrepancy between a person's actual bite and the way their jaw moves. The resulting jaw displacement causes their jaw muscles to tighten up during sleep, and it's this scenario that ultimately triggers the start of teeth clenching or grinding. If that abnormal pressure isn't treated, it begins to wear away the edges of a person's teeth and the protective, armor-like enamel that's meant to protect the soft dentin inside. Two signs that may have already happened is tooth sensitivity to hot or cold and cracks or lines appearing on the teeth. Another indication of bruxism damage is that pockets or notches called "abfractions" will form on a person's teeth, right at their gumline. But all of these issues are obviously just symptoms of an underlying problem that needs to be remedied as soon as possible.

Getting braces is often an essential first step to resolving the abnormal bite and tooth alignment issues that lead to tooth grinding. Creating a better bite with more even, spread-out pressure points relieves stress at the TMJ joint and relaxes the tight jaw muscles that can trigger tooth-grinding episodes. So once your son's bite is fixed and his teeth come together in a proper position, his grinding symptoms should improve. But even after his braces treatment is finished and his bite is corrected, your orthodontist will need to fabricate a night guard your son can wear during sleep to further protect his teeth from nighttime grinding. This removable device looks like a smaller version of a mouth guard, and it's usually made for the upper teeth only. Wearing it at night will provide a thick acrylic cushion between his upper and lower teeth. Any residual tooth grinding he does at night will put pressure on this acrylic material instead of his teeth and protect them from any further wear and tear.

Although you can buy inexpensive one-size-fits-all night guards at a drugstore to save money, they won't fit very well, which means they'll be uncomfortable. And they're often made from a softer material that tends to make wearers chew on the guard itself— which defeats the original purpose for using it, especially if it makes someone with bruxism grind their teeth even more than usual. That's why I would advise you to choose the kind of night guard that's been custom fabricated through a dental lab.

Since your son grinds his teeth, one more thing to remember is that he won't be able to wear a night guard at the same time he's wearing braces during treatment. Typically, he'd have to wait until he was done with his braces before he could start wearing a night guard. But there is a way to circumvent that issue, and this is where Invisalign treatment may come in handy. Since Invisalign trays are shaped like a night guard (but with much less thickness), his teeth will be protected as the plastic aligner trays come between his opposing teeth and prevent them from grinding against each other. Although Invisalign trays won't be as effective as a typical night guard, they can be used as a temporary night guard until your son's braces treatment is finished. This is the reason I usually recommend Invisalign over braces when I see a patient with a tooth grinding habit.

86. After a little more than two years in braces, I just got my braces off. I'm excited to be finished, and my teeth are straight, but I'm not completely happy about how I look. I think my gums have changed and are covering too much of my teeth, and I'd like to have that fixed. Is there any way to do that?

Enlargement of the gums while wearing braces is a common occurrence. And it happens most frequently when a person with braces hasn't been brushing well enough over the course of their orthodontic treatment. This oversight causes plaque and food debris to build up around braces and can lead to the gum overgrowth you're seeing. This is a very typical scenario, since it's simply more difficult to brush your teeth with braces on. If that's the reason your gums have enlarged, the simple act of brushing thoroughly and flossing daily for a few weeks—in conjunction with a good dental cleaning—will allow the gums to shrink back naturally by themselves.

If poor dental hygiene wasn't the reason for your excessive gum formation, it might have happened as a result of your teeth moving together to close a tooth gap during orthodontic treatment. When teeth must be brought together to fix a space, the gums get shoved along too, and that gum tissue has to go somewhere. As the space is closed, the tissue gets driven outward by the teeth, and this can cause the gums to swell up a little. Another reason to consider is that some people naturally have more gum tissue than others, and you might have had more of it to begin with—before braces treatment even started—and you didn't really notice it until you had your teeth fixed. The gums above your individual teeth may be higher or lower too, which can create the overall appearance of an uneven gumline when you smile.

But whatever the cause or appearance of the gum enlargement you're concerned about, it's usually an easy problem to fix with a gum recontouring procedure that can remove any excess gum tissue quickly, easily, and painlessly. In fact, I do this common procedure on a routine basis in my own orthodontic practice because it's so effective resolving my patients' aesthetic concerns about how their gums look. The procedure doesn't require any needle anesthesia, and a simple topical gel is all that's needed to numb the gums beforehand. After the gel is applied, I use a tiny laser to gently reshape and sculpt the gumline as desired. And because the laser beam instantly cauterizes the gum tissue, there isn't even any bleeding!

87. Now that my braces are off, I was advised to have my wisdom teeth taken out, even though they're healthy, so my teeth will stay straight. I don't even know which teeth they are, and if they're not decayed, why would they have to be extracted?

Wisdom teeth are located in the very back of your upper and lower jaw, and they're often called third molars, because they are third in line behind your first and second molars. Surprisingly, most adults don't have them at all, and when they do, they either don't erupt above the gumline or they emerge only part way. Occasionally, some people between ages seventeen and twenty-one will have third molars that erupt fully, but that's not really a problem. And despite what many people think, those wisdom teeth won't actually cause the kind of tooth crowding that will result in the misalignment of their teeth. That's really just a myth, because the forces exerted by the emergence of wisdom teeth are so small that they aren't able to move teeth and should not cause your teeth to shift at all. When people who had their wisdom teeth removed were compared with those who had not, there wasn't any difference in the amount their teeth had shifted after their braces were removed. It's like a game of tug-of-war where a solitary person has one end of the rope and is pulling against a big crowd on the other end. Who is going to exert more force?

Even though your wisdom teeth aren't hurting your new post-braces alignment, most orthodontists don't think wisdom teeth serve any useful purpose, and if they find any reason to remove them, they're definitely going to advise you to do that. One of the reasons your third molars might need to be removed is if they've only partially erupted—a common occurrence that promotes gum infection and tooth decay when food and bacteria collect in the gum flap that forms around them. So in cases where wisdom teeth are partially erupted, they're typically removed, even if the teeth themselves are healthy. But in situations where a person's wisdom teeth haven't emerged at all, and there's absolutely no possibility they could do so, whether to remove them should be assessed on a case-by-case basis. As an orthodontist myself, I can confidently tell you it never hurts to get a second specialist's opinion about the need to have your wisdom teeth removed. That's why I would typically refer you to an oral surgeon (who specializes in removing wisdom teeth) and let them make the decision.

88. When my orthodontist prescribed Invisalign therapy, he advised I use remote Dental Monitoring because I'm a nurse who has little time off. Can you explain how remote monitoring works and how it will help me while I'm getting my teeth fixed with Invisalign?

Since remote Dental Monitoring takes the place of in-office visits, many unnecessary appointments can be avoided, and a patient with a high-pressure job can spend less time traveling to their orthodontist's office. In other words, busy professionals like yourself can get the orthodontic treatment they need in a way that's more efficient for them. Dental Monitoring is a new technology that allows your orthodontist to check the position of your teeth wherever you are, once you've downloaded the Dental Monitoring app to your Android or Apple smartphone. And the way it works is surprisingly easy. Once you've started your Invisalign therapy and have begun wearing your clear aligners, you simply take a real-time photo and video of your teeth using your smartphone and then "scan" your teeth using the Dental Monitoring app. The images are uploaded to a computer server and monitored by an AI-driven computer algorithm and your orthodontist. These 3D scans are compared to your previous scans and to the incremental tooth shifting requirements of your ongoing Invisalign plan. Using this approach, we can accurately track whether your teeth are progressing according to that plan in a way that is most convenient for busy professionals who find it difficult to come in for appointments. Because some of my patients are coming from Ohio, Florida, and California, I've also found remote Dental Monitoring works well for people who travel a lot, either for business or pleasure.

What that means is my patients no longer have to postpone vacation plans or family visits or worry about how to schedule their orthodontic appointments around their business trips. By using remote Dental Monitoring, a patient's progress can be monitored from anywhere they're able to use the app on their smartphone, and my responses and recommendations can reach them wherever they happen to be. If one of my patients is wearing Invisalign tray number five, for instance, and remote monitoring shows me that tray's not adjusting their teeth as quickly as planned, I'll advise the patient to stay on tray number five for an additional week. Or if a patient feels some of their teeth are moving in a strange direction, they can use the app to send images and immediately communicate their concerns to me so I can evaluate their teeth remotely. The remote aspect of Dental Monitoring technology is very useful for patients with conventional braces too. If a patient is away at college and breaks a part of their braces, has a wire sticking out, or gets a sports injury and needs some advice, I can remotely view their problem and tell them what to do.

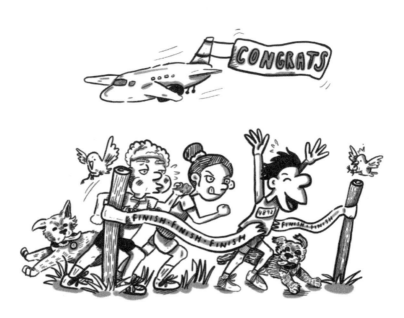

POST-BRACES: WHAT TO EXPECT

O nce your braces have been removed, the sight of your new smile in the mirror might convince you that you're all done fixing your teeth—but that's not the case. Caring for your teeth is a lifelong process. And even though completing orthodontic treatment ensures your teeth look and function much better, it's up to you to make certain they stay that way. During the initial days, weeks, and months after your braces first come off, your teeth will go through a post-braces adjustment period as they adapt and settle into their new positions. Some symptoms of this acclimation process—like the small calluses left by metal braces rubbing on the inside of the lips—will go away by themselves in a week. And the extra tooth and gum sensitivity you are likely to feel will disappear after a few days too. Until it does, it's best to resist the impulse to binge on all the crunchy and chewy foods you skipped while wearing your braces. This temporary residual tooth sensitivity is also the reason it's a good idea to avoid using tooth-whitening products for a month or two, even if your teeth look a little yellow. And because it is harder to keep your teeth and gums clean while wearing braces, you should have a dental exam shortly after your braces treatment ends to make sure you haven't developed any tooth decay or gum issues. All those guidelines are important, of course, but the most critical one is to wear your custom retainer to keep your teeth aligned properly. Although it's common to see your teeth move a little bit after your braces are taken off, wearing your retainer will ensure your teeth don't shift back to the way they were before you got braces.

---

89. What exactly is a retainer, and why will I have to wear one? I'm a high school senior who's just graduated and had my braces taken off. I wanted to be finished with wearing braces before I start college next fall, but now I've been told I'll have to wear a retainer. Are there different types of retainers with different benefits? Which one is best?

A retainer is a custom-made device you will wear after your braces are removed to retain the new alignment of your teeth—keeping them straight and in place—while your teeth settle into their new positions. Depending on which type you choose, you will eventually need to wear your retainer only at night while you sleep, so your new college friends won't even know you had braces unless you tell them. Your orthodontist can recommend which of the three basic types of retainers will suit you best, depending on your individual needs and how consistently you are keeping a daily routine. Among the three kinds of retainers, two types are removable, and a third is permanently (and conveniently) fixed in place to ensure newly

POST-BRACES: WHAT TO EXPECT

aligned teeth stay straight without you having to remember to take your retainer out and put it back in at set times. This permanent type of retainer is virtually invisible because it relies on a small wire glued to the back of the teeth (usually behind the lower front six teeth). And because this retainer stays on the teeth all the time, it can't get lost or forgotten. That might sound appealing, but when choosing a retainer, many of my patients prefer the removable kind made of clear plastic that fits comfortably over their teeth like Invisalign trays. The other alternative is to use a removable Hawley retainer that's more durable but bulkier, since it has an acrylic section that fits into the roof of the mouth. This retainer is also more noticeable when it's worn because the metal wires it relies on to hold the teeth in place will be visible across the front of your teeth.

90. As a busy working mom, I don't have time to research the pros and cons of which retainer is best for my teen who is about to get her braces off. Since there are different types of retainers, which one should I get for my daughter and why?

Most of my patients choose to get removable clear plastic retainers because they're the most visually appealing and comfortable to wear. When worn properly, they also work the most effectively at keeping your teeth from shifting out of alignment. So picking them as your retainer of choice would seem like a no-brainer. But they do have one drawback: they're simply not as durable as the Hawley type and will have to be replaced more frequently. Hawley retainers are sturdier than the clear kind, and I have seen them last over ten years. But the downside to these retainers is that they're more bulky and will cover your upper palate—which can trigger a gag reflex in some people. And

145

since Hawley retainers do not touch, or cover, every single one of your teeth, you run the risk of some minor shifting in your front teeth, even when you're wearing the retainer properly. They're also the most visible of the different retainer types, and when you're wearing one, you'll have a metal band running across the front of your upper and lower teeth.

The third type of retainer is called a fixed retainer, and it relies on wires placed behind your teeth to keep your teeth in alignment. These are typically used by people who, before treatment, have a severe amount of crowding in their front teeth. Although a fixed-type retainer is usually bonded on the lower front teeth, they are sometimes placed on the upper teeth as well. The reason some patients prefer this kind of retainer is because it can't be seen behind the teeth, and it doesn't have to be taken out and put in daily. These fixed-type retainers will also keep newly aligned teeth from shifting, even when a regular removable retainer is not worn. The downside to this kind of retainer is that it's not easy to clean when you're brushing your teeth, and it's very difficult to floss properly while wearing it. As you might predict, this oral hygiene issue creates the potential for dental decay and gum disease. Another shortcoming to consider is that fixed retainers may eventually break, causing new teeth to shift before the breakage is discovered. Because of this, I don't tend to put permanent retainers on kids, especially those with poor oral hygiene, since doing so could increase the likelihood they will develop cavities and gum problems. But if adult patients request them, I typically bond these permanent retainers on the back of their lower front teeth only. It's my professional opinion, however, that the majority of the patients I see will receive the most benefit from a clear removable retainer. In addition to being comfortable, visually discreet, and easy to take care of, it does a really good job keeping teeth straight after braces come off.

POST-BRACES: WHAT TO EXPECT

91. Working as a computer programmer, I have a lot of deadlines, and I forgot to wear my retainer for two weeks while I was finishing a software project. Now I'm worried because I can see that my teeth have shifted, and my retainer is hard to get on and doesn't seem to fit like it used to. What should I do?

If you forget to wear your retainers for a few weeks, and your teeth haven't shifted a lot, you can try to wear your retainer more (full time), and your teeth may revert back to the original position in some cases. The retainers will almost work like a set of Invisalign trays. But if they do not fit at all (you see a large gap between retainers and teeth) or they hurt too much when wearing, you may just need to get a new set of retainers. By doing so as quickly as possible, you'll prevent your teeth from moving even farther out of alignment, and they won't get any worse. Having said that, it's important I point out that the new retainer set won't reverse, or improve, the current misalignment of your teeth. It's also important to note this is typically only the case when your bite is decent and you've only experienced some mild relapse.

If you want more improvement, you can always opt to get a special type of retainer called a spring aligner. This would be the least expensive option when attempting to restore the alignment of your teeth. The problem with a spring aligner retainer is that this device doesn't always work as desired, since it won't give me the same control over your tooth movement I have with braces. Another factor to consider is that the appliance is bulky, and compliance can be an issue since it has to be worn almost full time.

If a spring aligner doesn't work, you may have to get braces again, but you might not have to get a full set of braces. Instead, you could opt for wearing sectional braces for three to six months—on your front few teeth only—if the adjustment you need isn't that sizable. In this scenario, once your front teeth are corrected and your sectional braces treatment is finished, you would need to get a new retainer to keep them that way. As a last option, you can always choose to get Invisalign to reposition your shifted teeth. Although using Invisalign to straighten teeth has many advantages, it may not be the best choice in a situation where you're only trying to restore the alignment you'd previously achieved with braces. Using Invisalign will be the highest cost recovery option when you're trying to make a minor correction to your tooth alignment. But there *is* a type of limited Invisalign such as Invisalign Express 5 or 10, which can come with a much lower price tag. So don't forget to ask about it, since it may be the best solution for you.

92. My teenage son just got his braces off, but he seems confused about how to take care of his retainer. As a single dad, I don't want to have to micromanage this task, so I'd like to know what you consider the most important best-use retainer guidelines my son will need to follow when using his retainer at home and school. Are there precautions he will need to take that he should know about?

Everyone scoffs at the trite and implausible excuse that "my dog ate my homework," but in the case of retainers, it's often true! Since retainers will stay in your son's mouth for hours at a time, they will have a saliva-and-food smell that dogs find extremely attractive. That's why I'm not surprised when patients come in and tell me their dog treated their retainer like a new chew toy, swiping it and destroying it as soon as the patient put it down somewhere. So keeping a retainer well away from pets is an important guideline to follow if you don't want to see a retainer chewed to pieces. Obviously, the moral of the story is to have your son keep his retainer in its case whenever he's not wearing it.

That simple practice would also prevent retainers from being inadvertently thrown away—another common problem that requires retainer replacement. Of course, it's quite understandable how that happens since kids and adults have to take their removable retainers out of their mouths before eating meals. What often happens is that they wrap their retainers in napkins and put them on the table, then forget about them. After they finish eating, the napkins (along with the retainers) are thrown into the trash. I've had parents tell me they went back to their child's school cafeteria and rummaged through the trash to find their child's lost retainer. Although some of those search efforts were actually successful, I obviously don't think it's a good idea to wear retainers that have been lying in a trash can for a few hours. If you're like many parents, you might think they could be disinfected, and some have tried to sterilize their children's retainers by putting them in a pot of boiling water. But removable retainers are made of a plastic material that's ruined by heat, so trying to boil them will just cause them to warp and melt. That's why they should never be left inside a car during hot summer days when the temperature inside will get so high it can easily distort the retainers and damage them beyond repair.

$93.$ Now that I've had my clear retainers for about a year, I just noticed my retainer is cracking, especially in the back. Since it's hard to take time off from my job to see my orthodontist, I'd like to know if this is normal. Is it okay to keep using it? Or should I call my orthodontist and order a replacement retainer?

When a retainer is cracking in the back (without being stepped on or suffering some other kind of impact), it could be a sign you are grinding, or clenching, your teeth. Since a person typically grinds their teeth only during sleep, you may not even be aware you're doing it. And because clear retainers cover the biting surfaces of your teeth, tooth grinding will subject them to such strong pressure, the force will eventually damage plastic retainers. Even if you're grinding your teeth for only five to ten minutes a night, out of a seven- or eight-hour sleep cycle, that amount will still generate enough pressure to crack your retainer over time. In fact, tooth grinding exerts so much sustained pressure, it will subject your retainer (and your teeth) to a significant amount of wear and tear.

Of course, tooth grinding isn't the only thing that can damage your retainer. *Clenching* your teeth during sleep can too. The kind of abnormal clenching I'm referring to sometimes happens when you're undergoing periods of stress—and headaches and jaw pain are two telltale signs you may be experiencing this kind of jaw pressure while you're asleep. Regardless of which is the culprit—tooth grinding or clenching—you might save wear and tear on your retainers by asking your orthodontist about making a night guard for you to wear while you sleep. A night guard is essentially a much thicker version of a retainer, and the night guard will not only help your regular retainer last longer; it will also protect your teeth from the inevitable cracking and wearing down that occurs when you have a tooth grinding or clenching habit.

If the crack in your retainer isn't in the back at all—but located between your two front teeth when you're wearing your retainer—it

POST-BRACES: WHAT TO EXPECT

could indicate you are taking your retainer out in the wrong way. This kind of damage can happen if you habitually remove your retainer by using your fingernail to snap it off your teeth, applying pressure in just one place, instead of gently removing your retainer using several fingers at once. And because any slight cracking can change the way your retainer fits, it may no longer be able to keep your teeth straight. As a retainer crack widens, you may even notice your retainer feels loose, a clear sign it no longer fits the way it should to prevent your teeth from shifting. So cracks or chips in your retainer are a pretty obvious sign you need to get your retainer replaced as soon as possible. If you don't wait but call your orthodontist quickly, the original mold taken for your retainer can be replicated quickly and easily without another impression being taken.

94. How long will my retainers last? Since I live in a rural area an hour's drive from my orthodontist, I was wondering if I'll have to replace them anytime soon. Will I have to get new ones in the future, or can I keep using the ones I was just given when my braces were taken off?

How long your retainers last is obviously going to depend on how well you take care of them. If you care for them correctly, they may last several years or more. But even if you do everything you're supposed to, retainers will wear down over time, and you'll eventually need to get a replacement. Retainers are like eyeglasses. You might be able to use them for a long time, but if you're not

> Retainers are like eyeglasses. You might be able to use them for a long time, but if you're not careful, you could scratch, crack, or break them and need to get a new pair.

careful, you could scratch, crack, or break them and need to get a new pair. Fortunately, there won't be any periodic prescription changes for your teeth the way there are for your eyes, and you won't have to get new retainers the way you have to get new eyeglasses. As an adult, your teeth and jaw won't normally get bigger or smaller, and once formed, the size of your teeth won't change unless a tooth is injured or wears down or you get a new dental filling or crown. So your retainers should last for many a long year before they will have to be replaced.

What's key to the optimal longevity of your retainers is treating them as though they're something fragile that can break. Just because they are made of plastic doesn't mean they can't be cracked or broken. That's why you need to be gentle when you take your retainers in and out of your mouth. And you need to be careful not to sit or step on them after you do, something that won't happen if you keep your retainers in a case to protect them from physical damage. Of course, keeping your retainer trays clean is important too, because letting them stay full of plaque and food debris can cause those trays, and your own teeth, to deteriorate quickly. So be sure to use a toothbrush and retainer-cleaning product to clean them thoroughly once a day to preserve your retainers and the health of your teeth and gums.

Fortunately, keeping your retainers in good condition has never been easier. You can order retainer-cleaning products online (such as from Amazon), and if you use those routinely, your retainers will stay nice and shiny the way they should be. Here's a little secret that can save you time and expense in the future too: since you just finished your treatment and got your braces off, let your orthodontist know you'd be interested in getting a second set of retainers for a discounted fee. By making that request at the time your braces are removed, there's a good chance you'll be given a substantial discount if you opt to get a second pair. What's really important about having that second set of retainers is that the extra pair might prevent the possibility you'd need to get braces treatment a second time. The reason I say that is because one of the most common reasons a person ends up needing retreatment is because they lose or break their retainers, and they don't have one to wear while they're waiting to see their orthodontist or to request a replacement.

This scenario is actually a fairly frequent one. My patients come in telling me, "Not too long after you took my braces off, I lost my retainers, but I didn't have a chance to come back in to see you. Now I can tell my teeth have shifted, and I'm worried I'll need to get braces all over again." To prevent this costly and frustrating outcome, it's a good idea to plan ahead and get a set of backup retainers, so you'll have an extra replacement pair to wear right away to prevent any shifting of your teeth. Some orthodontic offices have a retainer insurance program where you can pay an upfront fee to get free retainers for the rest of your life, even if you didn't have your braces done at that practice. So it might be wise to ask about signing up for this kind of retainer program to avoid unexpected costs. And if you *do* lose your retainer, don't wait, but call your orthodontist right away about getting a replacement. Some practices can even provide those the same day. The reason the time element is so important is that going without your retainer for just a few nights can cause your teeth to shift so much, your original retainer won't fit you anymore.

95. I'm about to get married, and I was excited to have my braces taken off before the ceremony. But now I see white spots on my teeth, and I'm concerned since they weren't there before I got braces. What

are these discolorations, and why do I have them? Is there some way to make them go away quickly?

White spots sometimes form around braces if plaque has been allowed to build up around them during orthodontic treatment. These spots are the result of decalcification where residual bacteria and plaque have released acids that have eaten away tiny areas of your tooth enamel. And the most common reason they develop is failing to brush your teeth properly during the course of your orthodontic treatment. Unfortunately, these white spots are permanent, and there's no way to reverse them or undo the enamel damage they signify. Whitening your teeth won't remove them. The only way to fade these white spots is with microabrasion (done by a general dentist), which removes just a tiny amount of tooth enamel around them so they look less conspicuous. Two other options are to replace the white spots with tiny dental fillings, using a tooth-colored composite filling material, or by getting veneers or crowns. When discussing the problem of white spots on the teeth, it's important to keep in mind that not everyone has tooth enamel that's equally strong, and it's a good idea to assess the integrity of your enamel before getting braces to begin with. Some people have unusually weak enamel, called hypoplasia—because their tooth enamel didn't develop properly during early childhood—and it's a condition that can predispose them to tooth decay and white spots if they get braces.

96. Should I have my wisdom teeth removed? I had braces a few years ago, but now I think my lower front teeth are shifting forward. Could my wisdom teeth be the cause?

In my professional opinion, there's no cause-and-effect relationship between the presence of wisdom teeth and your teeth shifting out of alignment during the years after your orthodontic treatment. When comparing the teeth of post-braces patients, the incidence of teeth relapsing into misalignment is just about the same, whether or not they still have their wisdom teeth. Despite this fact, many people still believe their wisdom teeth can somehow cause the crowding of their other teeth after they are straightened—even though the force of wisdom teeth eruption isn't strong enough to push their teeth forward. In reality, the most common cause of teeth shifting after braces is actually failing to wear your retainers every day the way you're supposed to.

Although I do recommend my patients get their wisdom teeth removed around age eighteen or nineteen, I always defer that decision to oral surgeons. They may tell you it's best to allow your wisdom teeth to grow in naturally if you have enough room in your jaw. But if you're like most people, and your jaw isn't big enough to accommodate your wisdom teeth without causing the overcrowding of your other teeth, they'll probably need to be removed before they have the chance to emerge. When that doesn't happen, and wisdom teeth are allowed to partially erupt (only part of the tooth has emerged) in an overcrowded jaw, they can come in at an angle and cause food impaction and decay.

97. After I got married, I found out my husband didn't like me wearing my retainers at night. I can wear them when he's not around, but I'd prefer not to have to wear them at all. When can I stop wearing retainers?

Even though you've had your teeth straightened, your teeth will continue to move for the rest of your life. So if you want to guarantee that your teeth will remain aligned in exactly the same position they were when your braces were removed, you will need to continue wearing your retainer for years to come. That's because your teeth and jaw are composed of living tissue, just like any other part of your body, and they undergo change over time.

If you got plastic surgery to remove your laugh lines next to your mouth or to smooth out the crow's-feet wrinkles around your eyes, you wouldn't expect that to last a lifetime, would you? And you won't look the same five years from now, right? Even if a person just lost thirty pounds, I can't assume they will remain the same weight for the rest of their lives because that's going to depend on their food choices, lifestyle, and their individual anatomy and physiology. But if you were told that you just had to wear a special magic belt (like your retainer) that would ensure your body would remain lean for the rest of your life, you'd be happy to wear it, wouldn't you? That's what a retainer does for your teeth: it keeps them in line and "in shape." And if you want to keep your good bite and straight teeth for the rest of your life, you will need to wear your retainer for the rest of your life too.

That said, you will only have to wear your retainer full time for the first four to six months after your braces are taken off. After that, I typically tell my patients they'll just need to wear their retainers during the night, before gradually transitioning to wearing them every other night. So in case you didn't catch that—eight months or so after getting your braces off, you should be wearing your retainers every other night—for the rest of your life. When the children I see in my practice ask how long they'll have to wear their retainers, I jokingly tell them, "Oh, you just need to wear your retainer for the next twenty years because after that, you'll be too old to care about looking great." Or I suggest, "Just wear your retainer for the next fifteen-and-a-half years." If they ask, "Why fifteen-and-a-half years?" I tell them, "By that time, I should have retired, and if you come back to see me, someone else will be here to tell you to keep wearing your retainer. And you can be angry at them instead of me!" But all joking aside, if you don't think wearing your retainer every other night is something your husband will eventually get used to, you might look into getting a permanent retainer, which doesn't show and stays on all the time to keep your teeth aligned.

98. Does everyone need to wear retainers after they get their braces off, or am I a special case for some reason? My coworkers say my teeth look great, now that my teeth are fixed. But my orthodontist says I'll still need to wear a retainer. Is this really necessary, and if so, how long will I have to use it?

Retainers are worn to maintain the healthy new position of your teeth after your orthodontic treatment is finished. To keep your teeth aligned and straight, it's essential that you immediately start wearing your retainers once your braces come off. Typically, I'll tell you to wear your retainers full time for the first four to six months, then during the night, every night, for another two to four months. After that, you can eventually transition to wearing them every other night, *indefinitely*. And this crucial requirement doesn't just apply to you; it applies to absolutely everyone who's had braces. The reason is that,

> Typically, I'll tell you to wear your retainers full time for the first four to six months, then during the night, every night, for another two to four months. After that, you can eventually transition to wearing them every other night, *indefinitely*.

over time, the majority of people (80 percent) who've had braces will have their teeth shift out of alignment if they don't wear their retainers consistently. Although I'm not saying your teeth will go back to their original pre-braces position, you will inevitably see some shifting if you don't wear your retainers. You might argue with me, saying you've heard that the teeth of 10–20 percent of the people who get braces seem to remain relatively straight without wearing retainers, but you'll have no way of knowing whether you're one of those people. So wearing your retainer is the only way to keep your teeth looking the way they did when your braces first came off.

99. I understand why I have to wear a retainer, but the one I was given has metal bands and large, pink plastic sections. My friends wear smaller retainers that look like clear trays, so why did I get different ones? I've also heard about permanent retainers. What are they, and would they work better for me for some reason?

The two most common types of removable retainers are either the bulky Hawley retainers, like you have, or the clear tray-type Essix retainers that resemble Invisalign trays. Although Hawley retainers used to be the most common type worn, Essix retainers are far more popular nowadays. It's easy to understand why so many people prefer them. They're not only smaller and much less visible but are far more comfortable to wear. And they even work better at keeping the teeth aligned because they make contact with every single tooth. The downside to these clear retainers is that they're not nearly as durable and long lasting as Hawley retainers and may eventually need to be replaced. That's especially true if you play sports or tend to grind your teeth at night. Since the material they're made of is more fragile than the opaque acrylic used to construct the Hawley type, it's easier to break or crack them, and it's also more difficult to keep them sparkling clean without scratching them. Hawley retainers are made of a thicker, sturdier acrylic, and you can simply brush them with a toothbrush and toothpaste to keep them clean.

But even though Hawley retainers are easier to clean and more durable, they won't totally prevent your teeth from shifting, even when they're worn as instructed. That's why some people prefer to use another kind of permanent retainers, composed of small thin wires that are glued on the back of the teeth to keep them straight. They're usually glued to the lower front teeth, because those are the teeth most likely to shift. But the downside to wearing this kind of permanent retainer is a higher risk of cavities and gum issues because wearing them makes it harder to brush and floss your teeth properly. This is why fixed retainers aren't prescribed for anyone who might have brushing compliance issues. But your orthodontist will know how to advise you, since they've gotten to know you over the course of your treatment. You can always ask to try the clear Essix type if you want to wear the kind of retainers your friends have.

100. With myself and two kids in braces, I'm concerned about the cost of replacing our retainers once our treatments are done. How long are retainers supposed to last? I know we'll have to wear them long term, so can you tell me how to help my kids and me take care of them, so I don't have to replace them too frequently?

With proper care, a retainer should last four to ten years, depending on what kind it is. But even with the best of care, clear retainers tend to be less durable than the Hawley (metal wires and acrylic) type of retainers. Whichever kind you and your kids have, don't try to superglue them together if they crack or break, since your orthodontist is the only one who can repair or replace them in a way that ensures they're still aligning the teeth properly. It's best to encourage your kids (and yourself) to get into the habit of keeping your retainers in a retainer case whenever they're not actually in your mouths. In the same way you're careful to put your credit cards back into your wallet, it's necessary to get into the habit of putting retainers away too and not leave them lying around.

As an orthodontist, I've been handing out retainers (or replacing broken ones) for two decades, so I can testify to the fact that most of my patients lose or damage their retainers in one of two ways: (1) they remove their retainers before a meal, and instead of placing them in a case, they wrap them in napkins, and they get thrown into the trash by mistake when they're done eating; or (2) they leave their retainers out where their dog can reach them, and the dog chews them up. It's not hard to understand why. Since retainers are worn in your mouth, they smell of food and saliva in a way that's irresistible to dogs who won't hesitate to confiscate them.

On that note, keeping your retainers clean is obviously very important to avoid bad breath, dental decay, and gum disease. Retainers should be cleaned thoroughly every day, and there are retainer-cleaning products you can purchase that do a great job, especially for the clear tray-type retainers that scratch easily. But whatever way you choose to clean them, don't put retainers in hot water (or an automatic dishwasher) because their shape may get distorted (especially the clear types). Some orthodontists encourage their patients to keep a spare retainer on hand at all times, just in case one is damaged or lost. And some offer free retainer replacements for life. That's actually a pretty good idea since just a few days without wearing your retainers can allow your teeth to shift out of alignment. So be sure to ask your orthodontist if they offer any kind of similar plan.

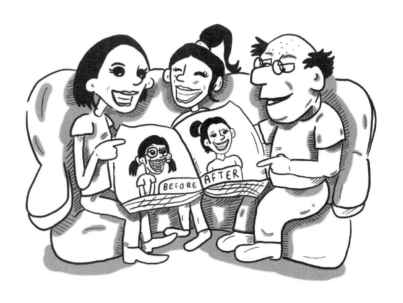

CHAPTER 9

SUCCESS STORIES

T he most amazing part of practicing orthodontics is getting to witness the gradual transformations of my patients—transformations that literally change their lives. As their smiles steadily improve over time, it's obvious to me that I'm doing far more than giving them healthy, well-functioning jaw alignments and straight teeth. Less noticeable, but just as important nonetheless, are the positive benefits to their mental attitudes and to their psychological and emotional well-being. As jaw pain is treated and resolved, for example, I see many of my patients cross over from depression to optimism—and as their smiles improve, they radiate a confidence that equips them to face the challenges of their lives in new and powerful ways. To show you what I mean, I'm sharing real accounts of orthodontic transformations I've overseen, only changing the names of the adults, teens, and kids whose anecdotes I've chosen to share. This sampling of patient success stories from my twenty years practicing orthodontics portrays only a few of the results I've achieved while treating under-bites, overbites, crossbites, crooked teeth, and extra or crowded teeth for patients across a wide spectrum of ages. By using the latest technology, avoiding tooth extractions, and offering complimentary laser treatment to reduce discomfort, I've been able to give my patients the kind of oral health many thought was impossible or out of reach for them financially. The following true success stories describe how I've been able to help a diverse array of patients achieve the proper symmetry of their jaws, faces, and smiles in a way that also helped resolve problems with their breathing, sleeping, and speaking. I hope these accounts will inspire you to wonder what this kind of treatment could do for you too!

Danny, an Eight-Year-Old Third Grader with an Overbite

When Danny's mom first brought her third-grade son in to be evaluated, I could immediately see he had a huge overjet (sometimes called an overbite). Not only were his top front teeth sticking out beyond his bottom teeth, but he had such a huge space between his front teeth, the other kids at school ridiculed him for it, calling him "SpongeBob." Kids can be very mean around this age, and it was quite understandable that he didn't want to attend school and cried every day about having to go. As a result of this high level of social stress, he was becoming more and more shy and withdrawn. By the time I saw Danny in my office, his mom was desperate for help. And I was very glad to be able to give it with phase-one orthodontic treatment. Danny wore a simple device to correct his jaw misalign-ment and a few braces to close the space between his front teeth—a course of treatment that lasted only about ten months. By the time it was finished, the change in Danny's personality was amazing. His mom watched in astonishment and gratitude as he went from a kid who was too shy to smile for photos to a boy who was beaming with confidence at school and eager to make new friends.

Jennifer, a Nineteen-Year-Old College Student with Severe Headaches

Jennifer was a college student who'd had previous orthodontic treatment a few years before she first came into my office with her mom for a consultation. They'd come in to see me because Jennifer was having such severe headaches, they were affecting her life in very serious ways. Her headaches had gotten so bad, she'd been forced to take a few semesters off from college just to manage her pain. Although she'd sought the help of many specialists before seeing me, including a neurologist and a physical therapist, none of them could help her. As a result, she was being heavily medicated to try to cope with the pain, but the side effects of her medicine made it impossible for her to study. Jennifer felt as though her life was falling apart, and she didn't know when she would be able to go back to school to finish her studies. Between her relentless headache pain and her inability to attend college, she became severely depressed.

When I examined her, I noticed right away that her bite was slightly off, but not to the degree that she would need braces all over again. Still, that was one indicator I found relevant. After some additional clinical testing, I noticed that her jaw's range of motion was limited and that her bite force was uneven, with some spots exerting unusually heavy pressure. Based on these findings, I recommended TruDenta therapy to try to relax any muscle spasms that might be occurring as a result of her jaw's uneven bite force. I couldn't promise her relief, but since nothing else had worked for her, and she had no other options, she was ready to try anything. Although I was initially hopeful, I didn't see much improvement after her first three session of TruDenta therapy, but by the seventh session, she had actually experienced some relief. Better yet, by her tenth session, Jennifer noticed significant improvement and a reduction in the intensity and frequency of her painful episodic headaches. And by her fifteenth session, she was so much better, she was able to go back to normal living without having to depend on her medications or endure their many side effects. Jennifer and her mom were so relieved, they were in tears. They hadn't known whether it would ever be possible for her to resume a normal life and go back to college to finish her degree. It is this sort of lifesaving treatment, one person at a time, that makes me feel truly grateful I'm an orthodontist.

> Jennifer and her mom were so relieved, they were in tears. They hadn't known whether it would ever be possible for her to resume a normal life and go back to college to finish her degree.

Robert, a Fifty-Year-Old Father with Worn Teeth

Sometimes parents become motivated to fix their own orthodontic problems after taking care of their children's. That's exactly what happened when Robert brought his fourteen-year-old son to my office to have his braces removed, since the teen's treatment was finished. Seeing how much better his son's teeth looked and functioned, Robert became interested in getting treatment for himself. "Hey, Doc!" he said. "As long as I'm here, I was wondering, could you take a look at my teeth too?" Although he seemed a bit sheepish about asking me to check his own mouth, thinking (like most people) that orthodontics is only for the young, I was quite happy to do so. And after examining him, I was particularly glad he'd reached out for my professional opinion. I saw right away that his lower front teeth were severely worn down and found out that he'd been experiencing pain and sensitivity in those teeth for a long time. In addition, I learned he had serious temporomandibular joint (TMJ) issues that had been generating pain in his jaw joint for such a long time, he actually thought such pain was normal! When I told Robert I was confident both his issues could be resolved, he was very excited. Now that all his children had finished their braces treatment, he knew it was finally his turn. He particularly liked the fact that the Invisalign therapy I prescribed was nearly invisible to coworkers and was convenient and comfortable to wear.

Over the course of his treatment, I heard a lot about how much his kids enjoyed teasing him on the issue of whether he'd remembered to put his trays in their case before he ate (as he'd reminded them so often), but the outcome of his treatment was excellent. Not only was I able to correct Robert's overbite that had caused so much damage to his lower teeth; I was able to successfully address his TMJ issues as well. I'd discovered that problem was the result of bruxism linked to the misalignment (overbite) of his jaw. To prevent any further damage to his teeth, I created a custom night guard for him to wear so he wouldn't continue to grind his teeth down while sleeping. Once his treatment was finished, his lower teeth were protected, and his TMJ symptoms were greatly reduced. Had his treatment been postponed, Robert would have eventually lost his lower teeth altogether.

Suyin, a Shy Thirty-Two-Year-Old Woman with Protruding Teeth

When I think about how orthodontic treatment can transform lives, I'm always happy to recall how it certainly did for a young woman named Suyin. She was thirty-two years old when she first came in to see me because she didn't like the appearance of her mouth and teeth. Right away I could see she had significant overcrowding and alignment issues that caused her mouth to flare out and her lips to protrude in an abnormal way. She seemed depressed because she thought her appearance was preventing her from achieving her life goals that included getting a new job, having a long-term relationship, and starting a family. Being self-conscious about her smile had made her very shy, and every time she laughed, she hid her mouth with her hands, so I wouldn't see how her teeth were sticking out and how enlarged her gums were. It was gratifying to let her know I could help her change those attributes with orthodontic treatment so she wouldn't feel the need to hide her smile.

To move her front teeth back, I prescribed braces and the removal of some of her overcrowded teeth. After Suyin's treatment was finished twenty-two months later, her face and profile were so drastically changed, she looked like a different person! It was almost as if she'd gotten plastic surgery. Her lips, which had previously stuck out so much she couldn't close her mouth, now looked completely normal. She was so thrilled with how she looked, she couldn't stop smiling, and she no longer tried to hide that smile behind her hand. I saw her back

> She was so thrilled with how she looked, she couldn't stop smiling, and she no longer tried to hide that smile behind her hand.

in my office two years later and was pleased to hear she had gotten the job she'd always wanted and was now married and had a child too. Of course, I can't prove that her orthodontic treatment and the transformation of her face led to her getting married and getting her dream job, but it certainly transformed her personality and attitude— two things that definitely helped.

Marjorie, a Forty-Five-Year-Old Lawyer with an Undiagnosed Condition

I was a little surprised when Marjorie came into my office for an initial consultation and immediately told me, "I want Invisalign so I can get my teeth fixed, and I want to start today!" As a forty-five-year-old attorney with a growing law practice, she obviously didn't have a problem with making up her mind. "Sure," I told her. "We can start your treatment right away, but first, we'll need to go ahead and take some x-rays." Since we always take cone beam computed tomography (CBCT) x-rays when first assessing patients, I was able to see a 3D rendering of Marjorie's jaw and tooth structures on images that were far more detailed than those produced by traditional panoramic x-rays—while exposing her to less radiation in the process. After obtaining the imaging and analyzing the data, I was startled by what I found. Her images showed dark-black areas where cysts were eating away the bone in her upper and lower jaws. I immediately referred her to an oral surgeon, who ordered a biopsy, then surgically removed the aggressive cysts. I'm thankful for the way Marjorie benefited from her 3D CBCT imaging since it was the diagnostic procedure that detected her abnormalities in time for them to be treated—something that wouldn't have been possible with traditional x-rays. If Marjorie had not come in for that initial consultation with me, or if we hadn't taken the 3D CBCT x-rays as we routinely do, I'm not sure what would have happened to her, since we would never have caught the cysts before they destroyed her jaw.

Liam, a Thirteen-Year-Old Boy with Long Incisors

Being self-conscious is fairly typical for thirteen-year-old boys, but I could tell Liam was more self-conscious than normal when he first came in for a consultation with his mom. After introducing myself, I asked him why he'd come to see me. Almost covering his mouth with his hands, which made it hard to hear him, Liam told me, "I have vampire teeth." I offered to take a look, and I saw that he did indeed have extralong canine incisors that stuck out on top of his other crooked and improperly positioned front teeth. He also seemed very nervous, and when I asked him if he was feeling anxious about anything, I found out the teenager thought his issues couldn't be corrected without having to pull a lot of his teeth. I assured him that wasn't the case and that we could definitely straighten his teeth without extracting a single tooth! He was very thankful to hear that braces could help him, and his look of relief was so dramatic, I couldn't help smiling. It reminded me that parents need to remember that many of their kids will resist getting braces because they've mistakenly assumed it's going to require tooth extractions. But just as in Liam's case, it usually doesn't, and he was happy to start treatment once he understood that. I was able to straighten his teeth and improve his jaw alignment so much, it even cleared up his speech issues by the time his braces treatment was completed. Thanks to getting treatment, he is now a beaming, confident teenage boy who speaks clearly and doesn't try to hide his smile behind his hands anymore.

Emma, an Eight-Year-Old Mouth Breather with a Crossbite

Only eight years old when I first met her, Emma was referred to me by her dentist because she had a serious crossbite. Her upper jaw was very narrow, and it looked as though it was shifting sideways every time she tried to bring her upper and lower teeth together. Besides the crooked appearance of her mismatched jaws, her crossbite created functional problems too, making it difficult for her to chew properly since the biting surfaces of her upper and lower teeth weren't meeting in the correct way to exert the degree of force needed. I could also see that she was a mouth breather, and her mother confirmed that, telling me Emma always kept her mouth open because she had so much difficulty breathing through her nose. When I looked at her x-rays, I could see why. The images showed her narrow upper jaw was restricting her airway in a way that had to be affecting her daytime breathing habits and causing obstructive sleep apnea issues as well. Now I understood why Emma's mother had reported the little girl hadn't been sleeping soundly—that she'd been snoring and waking herself up or having night terrors that made her afraid to go back to sleep. Emma's images also showed that her upper canines were coming in at an angle that could damage her front teeth, and I knew she needed immediate help.

I prescribed phase-one treatment to resolve Emma's crossbite using a simple palatal expander device she could wear in the roof of her mouth to gradually widen her upper jaw nonsurgically. I also advised Emma's mother to arrange to have her daughter's adenoids and tonsils removed to help resolve her sleep apnea. Thanks to these measures, I'm happy to report that Emma was able to start breathing through her nose, and her sleep improved after her early-phase orthodontic treatment. And when she got older, she didn't need to have braces of any kind because wearing her expander early created more space in her jaw, allowing her upper canines to come in properly without injuring the neighboring teeth around them. Most people don't realize that early orthodontic treatment with an expander can be a truly life-changing treatment, helping people chew, breathe, and sleep better for the rest of their lives. So many adult patients who suffer from sleep apnea could have been helped by using a simple expander like Emma did.

Oliver, a Seven-Year-Old Boy with an Underbite

As soon as seven-year-old Oliver walked into my office with his father for an evaluation, I could tell just by looking at him that he had the classic bulldog-like jaw that characterizes an underbite. His upper jaw was obviously too small, because his lower jaw was jutting out way beyond it. Like his jaws, his lower teeth were sticking out more than his upper teeth, and this gave Oliver's face an atypical, concave profile. When left uncorrected, an underbite inevitably results in abnormal tooth wearing, because the teeth of the upper and lower jaw don't interact properly. To remedy this, I began his phase-one treatment by fitting him with an expander device and prescribing face mask therapy. He had to wear the face mask only at night, but the expander needed to be worn in his upper palate full time. Using this approach, I was able to bring his upper jaw forward and successfully modify his jaw nonsurgically. This is possible only at an early age before the sutures, or growth plates, in a child's upper jaws have fused during puberty. Thanks to Oliver's vigilant parents, I was able to catch his problems at the right time, and together, we were able to address the bite issues that would have caused him a lifetime of orthodontic problems. If his underbite hadn't been treated before puberty like it was, the only way to correct it at a later time would have been through jaw surgery. Once his treatment was finished, Oliver no longer had the underbite that had created his concave profile, and his upper teeth were positioned slightly in front of his lower teeth in a normal way.

Amelia, a Fifty-Four-Year-Old Widow with a Narrow Smile

It was her birthday, and Amelia had just turned fifty-four years old when she first came to see me for a consultation. Since she wanted to begin a new phase of her life, starting orthodontic treatment was her birthday present to herself. Her husband had passed away five years before, and she was hoping to marry again and find someone who enjoyed traveling as much as she did. Amelia was still quite physically fit and moved gracefully like someone much younger, but when she looked in the mirror, she didn't like the look of her smile. Because her back teeth were narrow, there was a sizable dark space inside the corners of her mouth when she smiled, and that was compounded by the fact that her front teeth were angled in too much, making her look older than she actually was. I knew right away she was a perfect candidate for Damon Braces in combination with SureSmile. This combined approach successfully moved the angle of her upper teeth forward, making her smile wider and giving her lips more fullness. Once her back teeth were widened too, Amelia had a much broader, more engaging smile that made her look far more youthful. She was elated with the results of her treatment that took just eighteen months to complete. During that time, she'd planned her travel itinerary and started dating again and was having the time of her life. I was very pleased to have been part of her transformation, and Amelia was so grateful for her new youthful appearance, she still sends me Christmas cards with photos of her most recent travel adventures.

ABOUT THE AUTHOR

Christopher H. Chung graduated from UCLA in 1993, UCLA School of Dentistry in 1997, and University of Medicine and Dentistry of New Jersey (now Rutgers University) in 2000. He is a Roth/Williams-trained orthodontist and Invisalign Platinum provider who has been named a Top Dentist by *New Jersey Monthly* for the last ten years in a row.

Dr. Chung believes in the relentless pursuit to improve, because learning is never ending. Change is inevitable and requires that we constantly innovate and improve.

Dr. Chung is married with two daughters and a Balinese cat named Kipper. He lives in Bergen County, New Jersey.

OUR SERVICES

We have three practices in New Jersey, located in Millburn, Edison, and Union. Our practice has treated over six thousand patients over the course of twenty years. We focus on providing the highest-quality care using cutting-edge technology, offering 3D cone beam computed tomography x-rays with low radiation, iTero impression-less scanning, customized braces using SureSmile and Insignia, accelerated treatment, and Invisalign for teens and adults.

We believe in customer-centered care and always ask the question, "What makes great performance from patients' perspectives?" We want to wow our patients and deliver service that is second to none and more than what was promised.

Our mission statement is "to provide the world-class, five-star service that is second to none and patient-centered in everything we do." We understand that it's not about us but about the patients. We are not happy with just satisfied customers but rather strive for patients who are wowed and become raving fans.

Visit us at wowbraces.com.